AF757986

The Applied Anthropology of Obesity

The Applied Anthropology of Obesity

Prevention, Intervention, and Identity

Edited by
Chad T. Morris and Alexandra G. Lancey

LEXINGTON BOOKS
Lanham • Boulder • New York • London

Published by Lexington Books
An imprint of The Rowman & Littlefield Publishing Group, Inc.
4501 Forbes Boulevard, Suite 200, Lanham, Maryland 20706
www.rowman.com

Unit A, Whitacre Mews, 26-34 Stannary Street, London SE11 4AB

Copyright © 2015 by Lexington Books

All rights reserved. No part of this book may be reproduced in any form or by any electronic or mechanical means, including information storage and retrieval systems, without written permission from the publisher, except by a reviewer who may quote passages in a review.

British Library Cataloguing in Publication Information Available

Library of Congress Cataloging-in-Publication Data

Names: Morris, Chad T., editor. | Lancey, Alexandra G., editor.
Title: The applied anthropology of obesity : prevention, intervention, and identity / edited by Chad T. Morris and Alexandra G. Lancey.
Description: Lanham : Lexington Books, [2015] | Includes bibliographical references and index.
Identifiers: LCCN 2015039398| ISBN 9781498512633 (cloth : alk. paper) | ISBN 9781498512640 (electronic)

Subjects: LCSH: Obesity—Prevention. | Obesity—Social aspects—Research.
Classification: LCC RA645.O23 A67 2015 | DDC 362.1963/98—dc23 LC record available at http://lccn.loc.gov/2015039398

∞™ The paper used in this publication meets the minimum requirements of American National Standard for Information Sciences—Permanence of Paper for Printed Library Materials, ANSI/NISO Z39.48-1992.

Printed in the United States of America

Contents

List of Figures, Text Boxes & Tables

FIGURES

TEXT BOXES

TABLES

Acknowledgments

This book emerged from our desire to learn more about anthropological work in obesity, and particularly a wish to have a compendium of solid ideas for consideration in our own obesity prevention efforts. We were quite pleased to discover a large number of anthropologists devoting tremendous time, energy and expertise to issues of obesity, and have been inspired by how the many facets of that work reflect both the complexity of the obesity issue and the holistic nature of the anthropological endeavor. We are grateful to these authors for their dedication and knowledge and to Amy King and Francinia Williams at Lexington Books for their guidance. Morris further acknowledges the work of the many outstanding students and colleagues at Roanoke College whose energy and ideas have made his public health research not only possible, but fulfilling. He is also grateful to Emily, Ryan and Evan for the endless support and hope that they bring. Lancey is grateful for the opportunity to work on and learn from such a worthwhile volume with Dr. Morris, and for the guidance and knowledge of the generous faculty at both Roanoke College and the University of South Florida. She would also like to thank her friends, family, and her husband, Marshall, for their continued support.

Introduction

Chad T. Morris and Alexandra G. Lancey

On May 26, 1959, the American Heart Association held a "Symposium on the Prevention of Obesity" at the New York Academy of Medicine. The focus of the gathering was largely clinical, including presentations on genetics, diet planning, and pathology (Mayer 1960; Schur 1960; Hartroft 1960). One of the invited presenters, however, was a scholar whose work, by her own admission, was not in the realm of obesity at all. Hortense Powdermaker was an anthropologist who studied under Bronislaw Malinowski, and who is perhaps best known today for her ethnographic work in the Hollywood film industry (Cherneff and Hochwald 2006). Her remarks to the assembled experts in New York City that day, however, were discussions of the critical role of cultural norms, ritual and identity surrounding the acquisition, consumption, and provision of food in both the developed world and in what were then termed "primitive" societies: "The function of food and eating was, and still is, not restricted to the biological aspects. Food is the center of a complex value system and an elaborate ideology centers about it. Religious beliefs, rituals, prestige systems, etiquette, social organization, and group unity are related to food" (Powdermaker 1960, 287). She noted rising obesity prevalence despite improvements in public knowledge about nutrition, stating: "We ask, then, what cultural and psychological factors might be counteracting the effective work of nutritionists, physicians, beauty specialists, and advertisements in the mass media?" (Powdermaker 1960, 291). Well over 50 years later, the anthropologists who have contributed to this volume are still motivated by Powdermaker's question. Despite decades of public health effort, why does global obesity prevalence continue to rise? How can the anthropological endeavor lead to improved understanding of nutrition-related behavior, and what trials, ideas and successes can be shared by those who have sought to engage in the applied anthropology of obesity?

As Powdermaker surmised, increasing global prevalence of nutrition-based non-communicable disease is indeed a complicated phenomenon inclusive of many different causative factors, including food availability; social norms as evidenced in local foodways; genetic predisposition; economic circumstance; cultural variation in norms surrounding body composition; and policies affecting production, distribution and consumption of food locally and globally. The terminology surrounding these issues alone is quite diverse—"obesity," "metabolic syndrome," "food insecurity," "fat," "overweight," "food sovereignty," "overnutrition," "NCD"—and indicative of an important emerging area of study. Just as much work is being conducted to improve our understanding of these causative factors, there are also anthropologists working to find new ways to mitigate them. Academic contributions to the global issue of obesity have increased over the past decade, but so, too, has the amount of community-based work done by applied anthropologists whose efforts are more likely to be outlined in grant reports and presentations to community agencies than in academic volumes. To showcase this work, thereby advancing knowledge of obesity prevention, intervention and identity, we developed this text with two goals in mind:

1. Improving our understanding of human identity associated with obesity/overweight and how said identity is affected by cultural norms, policy decisions, and perceptions of cultural change (e.g., Am I obese/overweight or not? What does that mean about the way I see myself and others see me? Why has prevalence of obesity/overweight increased? How is it problematized or made acceptable? How, if at all, should obesity/overweight be defined and controlled, individually and societally?), and
2. Demonstrating best practices for the application of anthropological skillsets to develop culturally-appropriate nutritional behavior change across multiple levels of analysis, from local programming to policy decisions at local and national levels (e.g., What methods and approaches have proven fruitful? How can these levels of analysis be most successfully linked? What ideas and models have inspired change, and what key barriers have arisen? Can comparisons be drawn between efforts to address overweight/obesity in different parts of the world?).

The anthropological study of obesity lends itself quite well to application, judging by the applied nature of much anthropological work done in this area over the past several years. In addition to soliciting explanatory models used by respondents in different cultures and situations, anthropologists find themselves on the front lines of public health and policy attempts at affecting behavioral change. As such, we thought it important to create a volume that is applied in focus, so that it may be of utility to scholars and practitioners in applied and medical anthropology, as well as of potential use to public/global health scholars and professionals.

We have constructed, then, a volume of 12 chapters that cover the two key areas identified above with clear experience and breadth. The volume is geographically diverse; authors describe primary research in Japan, St. Lucia, Palau, Brazil and Costa Rica, in addition to U.S.-based work in settings such as a large university, an elementary school, a bariatric surgical center, a Native American community, and two Latino immigrant communities. The volume is also, we believe, methodologically rich. The work includes a mixture of qualitative and quantitative approaches to improving our knowledge of obesity/overweight phenomena, risks, and solutions; and reaches across the lifespan, from assessing participation in school-based programs targeting Palauan and American elementary students to chronicling reaction to Japanese policies requiring metabolic syndrome screening for adults aged 40-74. Importantly, the chapters discuss work that varies in longevity, as well, from discussion of initial results of community-based participatory research endeavors to assessment of the importance of longitudinal research and networking in achieving strong community health promotion programming and policy-level change.

Acting on longstanding calls for anthropologists to acknowledge and work across societal power structures (Nader 1972) and between studies of biology and culture (Goodman and Leatherman 1998), the volume encompasses multiple levels of analysis. Some chapters focus on policy; others on local programs or clinical realities. Many chapters operate across levels of analysis, linking grassroots community interactions to institutional and policy change. The volume is also intentional in its inclusion of authors from diverse settings. Authors hail from academic institutions and from positions outside of academia. We have included student authors as well (including co-editor Lancey), owing to the quality of their work and the immensely positive example that such work sets for other anthropology and public health students. Finally, we've asked all contributing authors to clearly highlight lessons learned and likely best practices, sharing these strategies and tips in a manner that might be of maximum benefit to practitioners seeking to create positive, sustainable change relative to obesity. In sum, the knowledge shared in the volume is diverse and complex, with ideas that are designed to assist in navigating the many settings and issues that readers may encounter in their own efforts to address the obesity phenomenon.

For ease of reference, we've arranged the chapters in the volume geographically. The first set of chapters focuses on work done outside of the United States. Lancey's work in both the United States and the Republic of Palau advances Powdermaker's assertion of the value of a comparative approach (1960), and serves as a bridge between the international and the U.S.-based portions of the text.

The book begins in the Republic of Palau, as Morris and colleagues demonstrate how a research effort focused on achieving Palauan explanations of obesity causation shows those explanations to lie largely in processes of globalization and in the nation's transition to westernized work expectations. The authors show how Palauans see obesity as attached to westernization, generational change, change in gender roles, and the roles played by convenience-seeking and new technology. Then, they seek Palauan ideas for obesity prevention and intervention, many of which are clearly tied to Palauan cultural identity. The chapter concludes with a discussion of efforts inspired by the act of seeking explanatory models and ideas from Palauans, followed by discussion of the importance of longitudinal research and partnership development in applied community-based health research.

O'Brien Cherry and Serieux also look to cultural factors and economic transition as explanations for obesity and noncommunicable disease. Chapter 2 continues with the assumption that food, obesity, and noncommunicable diseases are culturally-bound and therefore perceived differently among different cultural groups. This particular study is centered in St. Lucia, a country in a period of notable transition. Using qualitative methods that emphasize a collaborative approach, such as photovoice, the authors use an ecological model of health to link individual, community, and macro-level factors that have contributed to increased prevalence of noncommunicable disease. They identify key factors such as changing diets, the high cost of food, and a shift in economic subsistence from agriculture to tourism/service, and urbanization. This chapter also discusses a rise in psychological and psychosocial distress as a result of these factors (and how food is often used to cope with these issues). The authors conclude with the implications of this research for the development of cultural and community-based lifestyle intervention strategies.

Economic transition from agriculture to tourism-based subsistence plays a major role in the changing nutritional habits of the inhabitants of Dao and colleagues' study site in Costa Rica, as well. Chapter 3 serves three key purposes: first, to examine the role of critical pedagogy and academic partnerships in community-based participatory research by discussing the efforts of an anthropological field school focusing on global and community health in the Monteverde Zone in Costa Rica. Second, the chapter reviews the effectiveness of community gardens in addressing food insecurity and the related dietary and nutritional deficiencies that follow. Finally, the chapter describes the development and construction of demonstration "Keyhole gardens" (a technique that allows home gardening in regions where gardening is a challenge) as a means of increasing access to fresh produce for residents of the Monteverde Zone.

Klein's chapter examines how Brazilian policy makers have responded to obesity prevention through a multi-faceted food and nutritional security paradigm rather than the disease/epidemic framework that often dominates the

Ship To:

AMZ ORDERS APTP
800 AVONDALE AVE
COLUMBUS, OH 43212-3473

Order ID: 112-4959892-4588258

Thank you for buying from CARICA LLC on Amazon Marketplace.

Shipping Address:	Order Date:	Thu, Sep 24, 2026
AMZ ORDERS APTP	Shipping Service:	Standard
800 AVONDALE AVE	Buyer Name:	Jasper
COLUMBUS, OH 43212-3473	Seller Name:	CARICA LLC

Quantity	Product Details	Unit price	Order Totals
1	**The Applied Anthropology of Obesity: Prevention, Intervention, and Identity [Hardcover] [2015] Morris, Chad T.; Lancey, Alexandra G.; Alfonso, Moya L.; Arias-Steele, Sara; Bissett, Emily; Borovoy, Amy; Bruna, Sean; Brewis, Alexandra; Carney, Constanza; Chavez, Jose B. Rosales; Cherry, Colleen O'Brien; Dao, Lillie; Eisenberg, Merrill; Everett, Margaret; Klein, Charles H.; Kuartei, Stevenson; Luque, John S.; Malik, Zuhra; Serieux, Elizabeth; Sobell, Stacy; Tarasenko, Yelena N.; Tecum, Alejandro; Trainer, Sarah; Williams, Deborah; Wolfe, Amanda; Womack, Sarah; Wutich, Amber** **SKU:** 05088 **ASIN:** 1498512631 **Condition:** Used - Acceptable	$53.59	**Item subtotal** $53.59 **Shipping total** $6.77 **Item total** **$60.36**

	Condition note: Shows signs of wear. The book may have visible wear on the corners and edges- On the text block, it has stains and scratches		

Grand total: $60.36

Returning your item:

Go to "Your Account" on Amazon.com, click "Your Orders" and then click the "seller profile" link for this order to get information about the return and refund policies that apply.

Visit https://www.amazon.com/returns to print a return shipping label. Please have your order ID ready.

Thanks for buying on Amazon Marketplace. To provide feedback for the seller please visit www.amazon.com/feedback. To contact the seller, go to Your Orders in Your Account. Click the seller's name under the appropriate product. Then, in the "Further Information" section, click "Contact the Seller."

discourse. Chapter 4 opens with a discussion of the governmental structures and financial mechanisms that support Brazilian programs surrounding food and nutritional security, and describes many of the key programs and policies Brazil has established, including Food and Nutritional Security Councils, national conferences held every four years, the introduction of the right to food security into the Brazilian constitution, support for small and middle-scale farmers (including a woman's agricultural collective), community-based food education programs, and articulation with social movements. As part of this description, Klein presents an in-depth ethnographic study of a popular, government-sponsored restaurant network that provides low cost, healthy meals to low-income Brazilians in communal settings. He explores the best practices and lessons learned from this community-based (but uniquely government-supported) initiative to simultaneously counter food insecurity and promote healthy eating.

In Chapter 5, Borovoy continues Klein's focus on national policy by examining the Japanese public health approach to metabolic syndrome. The chapter includes a valuable depiction of the nation's metabolic syndrome screening program, which is mandated as part of regular health screening protocols for all citizens between the ages of 40 and 74. Borovoy goes on to explain prevention and treatment efforts associates with the Japanese characterization of metabolic syndrome, as well as key conceptual differences between the focus on metabolic function in the Japanese context and the focus on obesity as in other public health efforts globally. A key contribution of Borovoy's chapter highlights the metabolic syndrome approach's viability in light of the cultural values associated with family, school, health care and workplaces in Japan, examining cultural norms that might be indicated in order for lifestyle-based prevention and intervention approaches, such as a focus on metabolic syndrome, to bear fruit.

Lancey's chapter serves as a transition between the global and U.S.-based foci of the volume. This chapter describes a cross-cultural comparative approach to analyzing school nutrition education efforts (in this case, in the Republic of Palau and the southeastern U.S.). In schools, especially, programs are designed and implemented in order to educate students about healthy eating, cooking, and positive nutritional behaviors. Through surveying parents and teachers, several key findings about school nutrition education programming emerge, including the importance of parent involvement in program and policy development (and the relationship between this involvement and perceived program efficacy). The author looks to how these efforts could be improved to better capitalize on parent involvement. Finally, Chapter 6 discusses the importance of a comparative approach as it stands today, along with the benefits and potential contributions to the discipline of anthropology and current community health efforts aimed at obesity and nutrition.

Luque and colleagues represent the first of the book's six fully-U.S.-based chapters, but with a decidedly transnational focus. Chapter 7 discusses efforts to address obesity and diabetes among Latino immigrant communities in Southeast Georgia. The authors share key demographic information about Latino obesity and NCD in the United States, then share the results of two interventions designed to reduce obesity prevalence in local Latino communities. The chapter allows for useful comparison between two intervention types, one community-based (a non-medical case management approach for people with type 2 diabetes) and one investigator-driven (a nutrition workshop intervention developed as part of a broader effort to increase rates of cervical cancer screening). Their suggestions of including bilingual/bicultural staff, developing programs in partnership with stakeholders, and sharing program findings with the community are highlighted in a way that clearly resonates with work described elsewhere in the volume.

A focus on Latino populations in the United States continues in Chapter 8, where Everett and colleagues describe efforts to enhance utilization and access to local food markets for Latino and low income individuals in communities west of Portland, Oregon. This chapter is of particular methodological interest as it shares the use of public participation GIS as part of a broader Community-Based Participatory Research approach. Researchers were able to show that persons in predominately Latino and low-income neighborhoods were less likely to be aware of or utilize their local farmers market, then design interventions that appealed to those groups. Moreover, the chapter explains efforts to encourage local Latino and low income populations to produce food to sell at farmers markets, thus providing helpful treatment of both food production and consumption in community-based efforts to improve nutritional offerings.

Chapter 9 addresses theory and practice regarding type 2 diabetes management and prevention at Ysleta del Sur Pueblo, a federally recognized American Indian tribe in El Paso, Texas. Bruna reconceptualizes "translational theory" by focusing on how health interventions have traditionally been understood within indigenous communities, and argues for an emerging model of communal prevention that relies on preexisting local cultural practices, tying them in the biomedical practices for the best efficacy in diabetes prevention and intervention. He provides an example of this emerging model by drawing on his ethnographic fieldwork among the Ysleta del Sur Pueblo tribe, explaining that because tribal practices such as religious community gardens, pilgrimages and dancing are already popular throughout the community, they have the potential to become successful components of wellness programs for diabetes and obesity prevention. The chapter concludes with considerations for future research using this emerging model and discusses policy considerations for integrating culturally-appropriate interventions with the efforts of indigenous leaders and community health staff.

The next two chapters in this volume focus primarily on identity and using ethnographic methods to shift the attention to understanding and describing the "obesity epidemic" from the perspective of those who are already obese. In Chapter 10, Trainer and colleagues review the current ethnographic literature in order to support their argument that there is insufficient representation of perspectives of obese people. They describe their efforts to conduct an ethnography of clinical populations (specifically, those who are considering bariatric surgery) as a means to reveal new ways to support people already profoundly affected by the powerful, negative social understandings of obesity. By placing this clinic-based study in the context of the broader study of the anthropology of obesity, the authors suggest that there are multiple reasons that anthropologists have avoided listening closely to the needs and concerns of those who are most obese: the social invisibility and stigma, the difficulties in accessing informants around a highly sensitive topic, and the level of discomfort the extremely obese body seems to provoke (even in academic and scientific environments). In light of these reasons, Trainer and colleagues provide a strong set of recommendations for an engaged anthropology of obesity that properly includes these voices moving forward.

Chapter 11 builds on these questions of identity and perspective by seeking to understand stigma and discrimination through the preferred (and unpreferred) terms used to talk about overweight and obese people. In a study with young adults on a college campus, Williams and colleagues recruit students to elicit a core list of commonly applied terms related to large bodies, then surveyed more students as to the acceptability of use of these terms in both clinical and everyday settings. They followed this with ethnographic interviews with individual students to assist with interpreting their findings. Operating under the assumption that effective prevention and intervention requires an understanding of how the labels we apply are used in a wider array of contexts, the authors discuss how and when certain terms are used and share recommendations that can be applied in anthropological and public health contexts.

We conclude the volume with a contribution from Merrill Eisenberg, whose long career in the public health promotion trenches has led her to a particularly valuable perspective on community-derived policy efforts being a product of long-term relationship-building. Chapter 12 is process-oriented, and begins with a solid discussion of factors contributing to increasingly obesogenic environments in American communities, transitioning into a Tuscon, Arizona case study of efforts at achieving change in local zoning laws in order to encourage urban agriculture, including chicken-keeping. The emergent tale of issues in the problem, policy and political streams may well resonate with readers who have worked in health policy, and is certainly important reading for those who would seek to create local policy change. The chapter provides a fitting conclusion to the volume by reminding readers that time and rapport are critical components of efforts at achieving change in both policy and individual nutritional behavior, and that these efforts are ongoing.

Chapter 1

"Modernization," Global Influence and Obesity Prevention in the Republic of Palau

Chad T. Morris, Amanda Wolfe,
Sarah Womack, and Stevenson Kuartei

"There is a big sickness in this place," explained the elderly man from his home in rural Palau. "You know who brought that here? The U.S. and the Japanese . . . Everybody making rules and regulations. Not the people who have a right on it." "Big sickness" is the term that the man used to characterize increased prevalence of obesity in Palau. His perception of the problem's cause is one that is mentioned less often in scholarly discourse than more clinical explanations of obesity causation and prevention, but one that is echoed by many of Palau's citizens. In truth, explanatory models associated with obesity and nutrition-related behavior are often tied to social and political realities. Anthropological studies of obesity have been influential in identifying these explanatory models, from highlighting evolutionary influences on food choice (Armelagos 2010) and the importance of differences in normative body image (Brewis et al. 2011) to building complex understandings of how recent changes in global food distribution influence nutrition-based non-communicable disease (Brown 1991, Gewirtz and Errington 2010). This body of work suggests clear value in the study of processes of globalization relative to obesity prevalence, as does recent evidence quantitatively linking obesity to processes of economic, political, and social globalization in low- and middle-income nations (Goryakin et al. 2015).

The recent social and political history of the Republic of Palau ("Palau" hereafter) leads to local explanations of obesity and nutrition-based non-communicable disease ("NCD" hereafter) that are rooted as much in tales of colonialism and globalization as they are in calorie counts and food availability. Understanding the complex factors contributing to Palau's obesogenic environment is particularly critical given the estimate that 58% of the adult population, and 33% of the population of school-aged children, is obese

(Kuartei 2011), and data indicating high household prevalence of hypertension (24.1%) and diabetes mellitus (22.4%) (Ichiho et al. 2013).

Indeed, Palau has experienced a noticeable increase in obesity prevalence among its population of 20,000 people. Labarthe and colleagues, studying Palauan nutrition for the U.S. Navy as part of Trust Territory oversight in the early 1970, strongly suggest "modernization" to be the source of Palau's nutrition concerns. They describe modernization as "a composite of interactions of numerous physical, biological and sociocultural processes" (1973, 161), shedding light on the complexity of Palau's obesity concern even four-plus decades ago. Contemporary scholarship might more generally identify Palau's concern under the aegis of the term "globalization," given the strong role of foreign influence as it emerged in Palau beginning in the late 1800s and continues to this day. We begin by sharing this history, then by sharing the themes that Palauans use to explain concerns about nutrition and food sovereignty in the small island nation. Finally, we demonstrate how anthropological efforts to better understand local explanatory models and ideas have led to public health intervention.

"EVERYBODY MAKING RULES AND REGULATIONS": THE HISTORICAL CONTEXT

Foreign influence in Palau dates back to 1885 with the arrival of Spanish colonizers, though evidence exists of limited Western contact about 100 years prior. The Spanish exerted minimal influence in Palau. Germany officially occupied the Micronesian archipelago in 1898, commencing the process of stripping the islands of valuable natural resources. The conclusion of World War I saw the administration of Palau ceded to Japan, which established colonial infrastructure, including governance, schools and medical care, while furthering removal of natural resources (Labarthe et al. 1973). During World War II, Allied advances led Japanese authorities to forcibly relocate many Palauans to the more urban state of Koror (away from ancestral farming and fishing grounds) and develop significant military infrastructure, including a runway on the Palauan island Peleliu, making the island a strategic part of the war in the Pacific. Allied victory in the Battle of Peleliu (September-November 1944) and subsequent American oversight in Palau resulted in the region's inclusion in the United Nations Trust Territory of the Pacific Islands, specifically under the administration of the U.S., in 1947 (Gayle 1996, Shuster 2009).

American post-war administration of Palau began to transition into independent Palauan statehood via the development and approval of a Compact of Free Association between Palau and the United States. The Compact specifies

American responsibility for military defense of Palau, as well as significant financial assistance (over $400 million between 1994 and 2009) intended to assist Palau in achieving economic self-sufficiency. In exchange, the United States is granted access to territory in Palau for strategic military purposes, in addition to supportive diplomatic relations. Local approval of the Compact and the Palauan Constitution led to international recognition of an independent Republic of Palau in 1994 (Shuster 2009). The road to independence in Palau was not without significant local conflict, however, on issues such as military presence of nuclear material, governance structure, and concerns about Palauan subservience to the U.S. and other nations. The Compact agreement, officially ratified in 1994, was subject to review in 2009. That review led to an agreement for Compact extension until 2024, including an additional $215.75 million in funding (Reed 2011). The extension, however, has yet to be ratified by the U.S. Congress. Regardless, American influence in Palau can be seen in many ways, including economic assistance, military protection (including the ability of Palauans to serve in the United States Armed forces), and favorable labor agreements (Shuster 2009). Many Palauans have spent time in the United States, and decades of American influence following Japanese oversight have furthered westernized concepts of the work day and upward mobility, a significant departure from the traditional subsistence agriculture and fishing-based Palauan cultural norms chronicled by anthropologist Augustin Krämer in 1919. Today, Palauan grocery stores are filled with imported convenience foods, and comparatively little subsistence-based fishing and gardening is done.

The last 130 years in Palau might best be described as a crucible of globalization. One of the outcomes of this period of great change in Palauan society is significant change in behavior related to nutrition. Labarthe and colleagues were among the first scholars to consider the role of what they termed “modernization” in dietary change in Palau (1973). They assessed nutrition using modernization as a key variable, using “such characteristics as number of automobiles, quality of housing, density of population, access to commercial food products, involvement with a cash economy, and exposure to mass media” (Labarthe et al. 1973, 171). Using these criteria they selected three Palauan study sites, ranked from least to most modern: Ngerchelong (a rural state at the northern tip of the island of Babeldaob, home to most of Palau’s 16 states), Peleliu (an island state located about an hour south of Koror by boat), and Koror (Palau’s most populous state) (Labarthe et al. 1973). Their findings, specifically that “Results analyzed with and without geographic groupings showed consistent associations between modernization and health-related factors, with the most modern area having the least desirable health attributes” (Labarthe et al. 1973:161) serve as a foundation for our present work in Palau, including the selection of study sites in Ngarchelong and Ngerbeched (a neighborhood within Koror suggested by Ministry of Health collaborators due to diversity of population and perceived fruitfulness of prospective nutrition-based public health programming).

Labarthe and colleagues used blood samples and body measurement to determine obesity rates and overall nutrition in the three study populations (1973). Just as scholarly understanding of modernization and globalization has progressed since the 1970s, so too has our understanding of biological factors potentially leading to increased obesity prevalence. One of the biological hypotheses most commonly cited in considerations of Micronesian obesity is the thrifty gene hypothesis, which theorizes a selectively advantageous genetic predisposition to fat storage in hunter-gathering populations exposed to periods of rapid feast and famine, such as those likely faced by the seafarers who were to become Palau's genetic ancestors (Neel 1962, Kuartei 2005). Thrifty gene theory is subject to some debate in genetics scholarship, however. Speakman, for instance, argues that such genetic propensity is more likely to be emergent from an absence of selection, combined with genetic drift (2008). Whatever the genetic explanation, it seems reasonable to conclude that there is a genetic component to Palauan tendencies toward fat storage.

Photographs taken in the late 1800s, however, depict large groups of Palauans who are far from obese (see book cover). A realized propensity for fat storage requires, of course, the presence of surplus dietary fat. In the case of Palau, we turn again to global influence as a source of this surplus, and of diminished activity rates. Each political occupation of Palau has seen diminished reliance on fishing and gardening and increased food importation. Palauan exports have become almost nonexistent as the nation's raw materials have been exhausted and its primary worth in the eyes of global powers is now perceived to be its location (both for tourism and for military significance). Increased access to food such as canned meat and fried chips, exacerbated by the decrease in physical activity associated with transition to westernized concepts of labor, would seem to be the trigger for the "thrifty gene." In short, Palau's recent history provides many possible explanations for the Palauan obesity and NCD problem.

Our longitudinal work on issues of nutrition in Palau began in 2010, when the first author entered into conversation with then-Minister of Health Stevenson Kuartei, M.D. and his associates at the Ministry. Minister Kuartei had revealed in a conversation a few years prior his strong concerns about rising rates of diabetes, heart disease and obesity in Palau, and his interest in bringing Palauan cultural values to bear on finding a solution to what he described as a clear and growing epidemic. In 2010 and 2011, we created a strategy for anthropological research in Palau designed to: (1) assess the current state of Palauan understanding and practice relative to food consumption; (2) identify local ideas and practices for dietary improvement; (3) identify local ideas and practices relative to localized subsistence; and (4) work with Palauan community leaders to create and implement strategies designed to achieve dietary improvement and increased local food production. This strategy is rooted in tenets of Community Coalition Action Theory (CCAT) (Butterfoss and Kegler 2009, Morris 2011) and contemporary anthropological utilization of Community-Based Participatory Research (CBPR) (Israel et al. 2003). Importantly, this sort of community-based work is best accomplished via long-term collaboration and relationship-building. A long-term perspective reflects the best suggestions of contemporary anthropological discourse on community-based research partnerships (Schensul 2005), and is particularly critical to maintaining relationships in a nation that is often the recipient of short-term, grant-inspired assistance that can seemingly be of greater benefit to researchers than to respondents.

Our work in Palau has been designed from the start as a long-term partnership, and has purposefully sought to build relationships with the many Palauan agencies and individuals who serve as key stakeholders. While this research is geographically similar to the work of Labarthe and colleagues, our goal as anthropologists is more rooted in understanding explanatory models than in quantifying the nutritional status of Palauans. To understand more about the factors influencing obesity and NCD, we first sought to learn more about what Palauans themselves see as the causes of change in diet and health. Understanding how Palauans explain the problem, then, allows the development of culturally-appropriate public health intervention.

METHODS

We designed interview and focus group instruments in consultation with Ministry of Health officials, Palau Community College Office of Extension, and representatives of Ulkerruil A Klengar (UAK—a community health group) to include questions about food consumption, food acquisition, perceived causes of dietary change in Palau, NCD concern, sources of health information, and ideas for change. Operating under approval from Palau Ministry of Health and Roanoke College Institutional Review Boards, plus traditional leaders in the study communities, 17 Roanoke College fieldworkers began work in May, 2012. Investigators began by mapping households in each study community, then using the maps to randomly select respondent households. Provided signed informed consent (forms available in both English and Palauan), a semi-structured interview (approximately 45 minutes long) was conducted, recorded using field notes and digital audio recording devices. The interview was conducted in English (a language spoken by the vast majority of the Palauan population). Researchers were assisted by nine community guides selected with guidance from contacts in the Office of Cooperative Research and Extension at Palau Community College and Palau Community Action Agency. Community guides received a modest stipend for their assistance in achieving full consent, gaining rapport, and interpreting Palauan phrases into English, as needed.

We conducted 54 interviews: 34 in Ngerbeched and 20 in Ngarchelong. The additional interviews in Ngerbeched are consistent with that community's larger population compared to that of Ngarchelong. In addition, two focus groups were conducted with community leaders and parents. The purpose of the focus groups was to provide group-derived data that individual interviews might miss, and to begin to form a framework for later community-based public health program design. Focus groups were around an hour in length, and were recorded using field notes and digital audio recording devices.

Interviews and focus groups were transcribed, coded, and analyzed using Nvivo software. What follows is presentation and discussion of the several Palauan explanations for the local rise in nutrition-based non-communicable disease prevalence, followed by an account of some of the early means by which this improved understanding of Palauan explanatory models has been put to use in applied efforts to reverse the NCD trend.

"YOU KNOW WHO BROUGHT THAT HERE?": EXPLANATIONS OF INCREASED OBESITY PREVALENCE

Palauan respondents demonstrated complex understanding of change in Palauan subsistence and nutrition over time, positing clear linkages between globalization and obesity and NCD prevalence. Nearly all respondents saw NCD as an important issue facing the people of Palau, though there was significant variation in operational knowledge and perceptions of NCD causation, consequence, and prevention. Explanations of increased obesity prevalence coalesced into four main themes: the role and influence of Westernization, change across generations, change in traditional gender roles, and discussion of technological convenience.

Westernization

Many respondents mentioned Westernization, and particularly American influence, in response to questions about reasons for change in subsistence and the rise of obesity and NCD. To some, including the gentleman whose remarks begin this chapter, the ties between foreign influence and nutritional change are so clear as to be causative. One pinpointed reason for Westernization-related changes is transition to a wage-earning system based on the U.S. Dollar, as opposed to traditional family, clan and village-based reciprocity as seen by Krämer (1919) and recounted to Johannes (1981). One respondent states: "But you know, you guys, you are American. You come in and teach us how to use dollar sign. That's why we go, we're looking for dollar. Every day. We wake up in the morning, I go to work, I earn as much money, never mind the farm. I buy with this much money, I go to the store and buy." Types of labor have changed over time in Palau, as well. Palauans point out that contemporary labor tends to be more sedentary, combining nutrition-based health concerns with broader concerns about changes in available food:

> My father, we all used to be before. We were tall, muscular, and strong because we always ate fresh food and we usually, at that time, no carbs. Very few. And when they go fishing, they all use bamboo rod. Prepared to go fishing. A lot of exercise. They do cut trees for building real fire. They, they move everything. And men, Western influence came in. They screw up everything, everything, all the food. Artificial food, some strong chemicals, the preservative. Those are poison.

Reliance on imported food has increased substantially in Palau, leading not only to concerns about nutrition, but also to concerns about food supply. For instance, a dockworker strike in California can cause Palauans to largely go without fresh vegetables and eggs for an extended period, to say nothing of the fear that natural disaster such as a typhoon might render Palau's single commercial shipping port inoperable.

While some respondents spoke of food availability, others spoke of a social premium being placed on Western food: "It's already changed. I recognize it. Young kids less like to fish and just like to go to restaurant and eat fast food. Pizza, burger. One of my nephews doesn't eat fish." In addition to American influence in Palau, respondents spoke of the effect of television and increased travel outside of Palau on changing dietary desires. A Palauan woman, speaking of her children, lamented: "they watch TV and they look at the food and they ask I'd like to try that one." Similarly, respondents spoke of increasing Palauan computer/internet/smartphone usage as a source of the Western influence that they associate with obesity.

Brown (1991) points out that the rapid spread of westernization does not increase the world's food supply nearly as much as it redistributes that supply. As scholars such as Gewertz and Errington (2010) and Singer (2014) have found in their study of food imports elsewhere in the Pacific, redistribution of the world's food supply to periphery nations tends to take the form of less nutritious, calorically dense food. In the case of Palau, it seems likely that overeating isn't so much a primary cause of obesity as is the replacement of traditional systems of subsistence with a wage-based system, itself necessitating replacement of locally-produced fresh foods with imported packaged, canned and frozen food of lesser nutritional quality.

Generational Change

Almost all respondents in the 2012 interviews recognized that even recent Palauan generations lived very different lifestyles than those seen in contemporary Palau. Several of these respondents saw lifestyle change across generations as a cause of health decline:

> My mom was a homemaker. She did taro patch; she has taro patch. And so, what our main diet was fish and taro. And fruits, we had a lot of local fruits we eat every day. That was like in between meals, is just fruits. Pineapple, local apples, starfruit, sugar cane, just chew on the sugar cane. Nowadays, it's not. I have to buy him snacks, and it's an apple or the gummy bears, fruity gummy things, yeah. Those things, I have to buy him those. Or, cereals. I just put cereals in a lunch sandwich bag. That would be his snack for school. Before, we didn't have those. We had to fix our own snack from a tree.

Respondents reported seeing and participating in much less farming and fishing than in the recent past, citing the change as occurring largely between the post-war years and the 1980s. Some parents claimed that their children show disinterest in wanting to learn traditional Palauan subsistence practice, raising alarm that key aspects of Palauan culture are quickly disappearing.

Some of the more elderly Palauans we spoke with had similar concerns. Others found hope, though, in the efforts of Palauan elementary schools to create school gardens, thereby introducing traditional foods and subsistence knowledge to Palauan children: "But at our school, Koror Elementary School, we have a farm that the third graders, fifth graders are responsible of. And that farm, has bananas, cucumbers, zucchini, you name it, they have it there. And they harvest green beans, and they harvest, and bring it to the kitchen, and the cook will cook it for the kids." Complaints and concerns regarding Palauan children, interestingly, aren't unlike those sometimes heard about American children. Palauan parents want their children to spend more time outside and eat healthier like they did when they were younger, yet express guilt that they fail to model the lifestyle they want their children to live: "We cook meat, yeah, we give them mayonnaise to eat, we buy corned beef. I think it's our fault." Some respondents expressed worry that Palauan children are developing NCDs early in their lives, with concomitant decrease in life expectancy: "It's a very big issue because a lot of people are getting diabetic, even younger people. I have a small cousin, only 8 years old and she is diabetic. I didn't know that that could hit a young kid that it's only like for old people like, over 40s. It's really a big wake-up call like this NCD thing is serious." "Epidemic" is a term that has been used to describe childhood obesity in Palau (Kuartei 2011). Moffat cautions that application of the term "epidemic" to increased childhood obesity prevalence is misleading as the term has more traditionally been applied to infectious disease outbreaks that have vastly different frameworks for prevention and intervention. Instead, she suggests viewing childhood obesity through a different lens, focusing not on immediacy of treatment, but rather on complexity of the social and environmental forces that shape both the problem and potential solutions (Moffat 2010). In the case of Palau, where there is indeed concern that increasing numbers of parents may outlive their children due to the rapid pace of dietary change and associated NCDs, there is clear need for the more complex framing that Moffat suggests.

While we didn't interview children in 2012 (we did so in 2015 field research in schools, now being analyzed), it seems worthwhile to mention concern about stigma surrounding childhood obesity. In generations past, high child body weight was seen as a sign of the parents' ability to provide for the child. As Palauans have been influenced by Western body image norms, Palauan children today face the challenge of growing up with the burden of an obesogenic environment combined with peer scrutiny. Given mixed nutritional messages for Palauan children and their parents, Palau is particularly predisposed to 'othering' in regards to body image, in which children (and their parents) tend to see themselves as normal in size (Taylor 2015). This phenomenon may further complicate efforts at treatment and prevention.

Gender Roles

Traditional Palauan gender roles in providing food for the family were split so that the men completed the fishing and the women farmed. Palau is a matrilineal society, and women's groups have long held political significance in local governance. It is perhaps not surprising, then, to see that Palauan women have quickly come to play a significant role in the Westernized workforce. Several respondents saw these changes in gender roles as part of Palau's obesity problem, particularly in terms of changes in food consumed. Respondents indicated that, especially for women, adoption of the American-style work week means less time to grow and catch for your own family and more money to buy food from the store:

> Today you hardly see people going out and gardening. And I think because our moms, they were stay at home moms they work at the house and do their garden, while today most mothers are working. And, I have three kids and I have

> a domestic helper. So then sometimes I'll come home and I'm too tired and she cook and clean the house and do the housework.

In addition to obesity concerns, Palauan parents and grandparents see the shift away from traditional roles as detrimental to Palauan identity both personally and nationally. The fruits of their labor are sources of pride for Palauans. As one Palauan woman noted, Palau is losing one of its historically defining characteristics: being the only nation in Micronesia where women rather than men traditionally farmed. Farming today is seen by many as done by "only the old people, 50 to 60 or 70, between the age of 50 to 70, those are the people that usually go to the garden. But not the young people." In fact, farming today conveys a different sort of social status in Palau, as the ability to afford agricultural labor on ancestral land is a sign of wealth: "I think part of the reason is that before it was . . . it had to be done. And people were doing it. And now it's only those who have money to hire people from Bangladesh or the Philippines just to fix the farm and taro patches." The commodification of subsistence crops is not a new global phenomenon, of course, but therein, as in many areas of Palauan life, we see particularly rapid change not only in purpose of farm labor, but also in gender roles as it is not uncommon for Palauan women to be primary wage earners in a household.

Subsistence fishing, traditionally the purview of males in Palau, has also declined substantially according to respondents, giving way to consumption of canned and frozen meat and fishing for profit. Reasons for the decline are tied both to work days and access to technology such as motorized boats and refrigeration: "When I was growing up it was the number of freezers and refrigerators was slimmer. So the way people go out and fish is just to get enough for them. But nowadays people go out and they get and sell or get more than what they need." The fish the men catch and the taro the women grow are indicative of their ability to provide in the minds of Palauans. Another Palauan commented that "it breaks their pride" when fish is purchased from the store "because it's Palauan men buying another man's fish," which is described as "not a good thing for Palau." In other words, at least some Palauans appear to view the shift away from traditional gender roles as demoralizing, particularly given nutritional consequences of the change. Younger generations are beginning to push beyond traditional gender roles, as evidenced by a young woman's statement: "Sometimes my grandpa says, 'let's go fishing.' I'm excited to go with him! And he say 'you're a girl, you don't have to go,' but I told my grandpa that it doesn't matter if you're a boy or a girl." Change in gender roles associated with subsistence is most certainly aligned with change in gender roles in other aspects of Palauan society, including governance. Female influence in traditional Palauan culture has long been strong enough to affect local decision-making or even strip a chief of his title. That influence remains today not only in relation to traditional leadership structures, but also in places like the Palauan senate (*Olbiil er a Kelulau*).

Convenience/Technology

Simply put, buying canned or frozen food from the grocery store is cheaper and easier than growing, catching, or even buying fresh foods in Palau, as is often the case worldwide. As noted above, many respondents pointed out that Westernized lifestyles and workdays leave little to no time for traditional Palauan subsistence strategies of growing and catching food. Respondents provided a substantial list of barriers associated with contemporary pursuit of the fishing and farming that were once much larger parts of Palauan identity.

Fishing, traditionally done by the males of the household and taught from an early age, has always been a large source for the Palauan diet for obvious reasons. Fishing canoes have given way to motorized boats, leaving Palauans to face the challenge of high fuel prices. With a national minimum wage of $3.00 per hour and fuel prices in excess of $5.00 per gallon, sufficient boat fuel for family subsistence is a major concern, as is time for fishing for those who have other jobs: "When I was growing up and we lived in Melekeok we lived by the beach. So every time we wanted to go fishing we would go out. It doesn't matter. But living here in Koror, if I want to go fishing, I either drive to Melekeok or I go with my brother on his boat and I have to buy gas. And I have to drive to the port." Large-scale and commercial fishing have the advantage of selling their catch to fund their fuel costs. Palauans often find themselves buying fish caught in their own waters, canned or frozen in another country, and sold back to Palau. Further, commercial fishing has greatly reduced fish stocks near shore, meaning that successful fishing excursions require more and more fuel to complete.

Another inconvenience associated with Palauan subsistence has to do with access to land. Many of the Palauan families who were forced to move to Koror during Japanese occupation never returned to ancestral land elsewhere in Palau. As such, respondents in urban Ngerbeched pointed out that land for gardening is scarce, and travel to family land elsewhere (if it exists and the location is known) is onerous. Farming and gardening have other costs too, of course, including time and materials. These costs, as noted above, have led agriculture in Palau to be seen today as an activity to be performed by foreign laborers.

Interestingly, many Palauans described the transition away from farming and fishing and toward more convenient means of food procurement as a form of culture-wide laziness: "If you are hungry and you are lazy, and you don't want to cook, just run to the store, buy corned beef, open it, and that's it. So it's about laziness." The laziness theme surfaced in the majority of the interviews, revealing widespread concerns about Palauan identity. To many, failure to farm or fish in the manner of the elders is expressed as a personal and cultural failing—laziness—that may well be serving as a barrier to meaningful dietary change. Above all else, the most common concern that respondents associate with modern Palauan life is that of busy-ness, particularly when Palau is placed in the sphere of contemporary nationhood: "I think that people are just so busy and getting busier because were a tiny country that's trying to do everything that a big country does. So everybody wears multiple hats. Doing so many different things." One respondent who had spent several years living in the United States compared life in Palau to life there, asserting that Palauan life is much more hectic, with much less free time. In this regard, it seems as though a Palauan propensity for convenience may be born of necessity. Regardless, many Palauans link dietary habits associated with the contemporary pace of life to obesity and NCD.

PALAUAN IDEAS FOR OBESITY PREVENTION

The causes of Palauan obesity and NCD, as stated by respondents in Ngerbeched and Ngarchelong, are rooted in largely recent changes in subsistence, economic system, governance, gender roles, and, of course, culture. The pace of these changes, magnified in Palau's small population, places the people of Palau squarely within a crucible of globalization. This crucible has produced, among other outcomes, a crisis of diseases—obesity, diabetes, cardiovascular disease—with which humanity has not long been familiar. What we do know, based on observations of other societies with similar concerns, is that changes in culture and identity associated with globalization cannot simply be shoved back into Pandora's box. Reversion to original patterns of subsistence and governance is no more welcome to most citizens of Palau than reversion to a time without penicillin or the internet. Palauan identity and behavior has changed with incredible speed, but there is evidence that positive change might occur with similar speed. The question facing us is how to guide the path forward to include more healthful behavior.

One of the key benefits of using community-based approaches to NCD prevention, such as CCAT and CBPR, can be found in the solicitation of locally-derived ideas for change. As Hyland notes, "No longer is it sufficient to enter a community setting, bring our expertise to bear on its problems, and then leave after attempting to resolve some of those problems. Rather, we must engage affected community members" (2005, 230). Palauans have been faced with no shortage of well-meaning but poorly adapted educational materials and program ideas from external experts. The present research is not in a position to determine efficacy of these efforts, but it seems clear that such efforts often fall short of engaging local cultural norms, explanatory models, and stated needs. Given the complex etiology of Palau's obesity concerns, we maintain that efforts to improve Palauan obesity rates should be better rooted in local ideas. As such, we asked two specific interview questions aimed at identifying Palauan ideas for change: "What would be the best way to encourage Palauans to grow or catch more of their own food" and "If you could make some changes in Palauan communities or policy aimed at improving nutrition, what would they be?" Responses to these questions fell into three main themes: education, community activities and policy.

Education

Many respondents believed that teaching children about gardening in schools would be beneficial. One respondent indicated that Koror Elementary School already had such a program in place: "Koror Elementary School, the school right above there, I think it's 6th grade or 7th graders. They have a gardening class which they grow tapioca." In the interviews, it was also expressed that children should be learning about the traditional Palauan foods in school. Importantly, schools are not the only source of education for Palauan children. Local comments reflect that they learn actively in the home, as well as via sports camps and teams and religious group gatherings, and suggest improved focus on nutrition education in these settings.

Adult education was also an idea that came up often during interviews. Many respondents suggested that seminars for the community have been helpful, convenient, and cost effective. Seminar topics from NCD education to cooking demonstrations were suggested. Also, during these seminars (or in separate marketing efforts), some respondents indicated that it would be beneficial to use examples of Palauans suffering from NCDs to help reiterate their point.

Community Activities

Community activities, from small gatherings of elder women, to in-home cooking demonstrations, to meetings at houses of worship, were commonly seen by respondents as potentially fruitful means of encouraging improved nutrition and encouraging local food production. Respondents said that while many people do not have time to garden on their own, people would be more likely to participate in community gardens. Respondents believed that having such spaces in each community would be beneficial. One respondent indicated that a good idea would be to:

> Bring everybody like, all the women in the little town here, get together every once a month and have like a big garden where they can grow all kinds of vegetables, and bring all the students in I guess, the more they see different kinds of vegetables, instead of just taro and tapioca, have like tomatoes, stuff like that so they can see a whole bunch . . . so the community . . . can come and pick their own food for free and bring it home, maybe that could help out and encourage the whole neighborhood to grow more. I think that's a good idea, you know, come on, let's go farming!

This type of community garden would allow Palauans to be more self-sustaining when it comes to food, though a few respondents saw the barrier of time as detrimental to a community garden idea. Another concern has to do with social status. As mentioned above, agriculture in contemporary Palau is seen by many as something that is done by elderly women, the poor, or foreign workers hired by wealthy land-owners. Several respondents suggested that efforts such as providing land for crop-tending (or encouraging gardening at home) would be more effective if focus was placed on sparking the creation of small groups of like-minded community members to support one another. Community-based women's groups have traditionally held great political and social significance in Palau's matrilineal society (Krämer 1919, Useem 1950), so it is not surprising to see Palauan respondents looking to such groups as important in establishing community gardening programs. In addition, school gardens are tended to some degree by parents and teachers from the surrounding community. All told, increased crop production was one of the most common ideas mentioned.

Policy

Finally, the Palauans interviewed expressed the need to change or create certain policies regarding health and nutrition. Specifically, many Palauans mentioned that there should be certain restrictions on imported foods, canned foods, cigarettes, and alcohol. A higher tax on canned foods was a suggestion made by more than a few respondents.

Importantly in the area of policy, respondents reminded us that the transition to new and at times parallel forms of governance has not been without its challenges. When asked who should run the nutrition seminars mentioned in the education section above, one respondent suggested against government officials: "I don't wanna just bring somebody that's gonna come here and, they're high officials but they don't have the heart for it." This is but one example of a clear government/community dichotomy that was pervasive in the interviews, and is worthy of further exploration. Many respondents seem to place more trust in community efforts to improve nutrition than in governmental efforts. At the same time, many respondents praise recent NCD awareness efforts undertaken by the Ministry of Health and others. As such, it seems evident that a community-based approach to reducing obesity rates, focusing specifically on inclusion of diverse community stakeholders across any perceived government/community divide, would be beneficial to citizens of Ngarchelong and Ngerbeched.

"A BIG SICKNESS IN THIS PLACE": TURNING RESEARCH INTO ACTION

Data analysis reveals a need and desire for nutrition education in Palau, particularly at the community level, while showing the great promise of leveraging Palauan identity in improving food availability and decision-making. The data also reveal that Palauans rightly have a complex understanding of NCD concerns as the product of the broader globalizing forces to which they have been subjected. Finally, it is abundantly clear that external influence that doesn't take Palau's history and culture into account (along the lines of "everybody making rules and regulations") is unlikely to be a viable solution to Palau's nutrition concerns. In fact, it may be more likely that Palauan ideas can be brought to bear in improving health not only in Palau, but potentially in other places where obesity prevalence is strongly tied to globalization. We conclude this chapter with a brief discussion of efforts spawned thus far by our research into Palauan explanations of obesity causation, alongside lessons that may be of broader relevance to the applied anthropology of obesity.

Conversation with government and community partners in Palau led our grant writing efforts to be focused on provision of nutrition related messaging through television, radio and nutrition workshops. It was also important to us that the messengers across each of these initiatives be Palauan, and that the messages offered be appropriately specific to Palauan traditions, places and cultural norms. Given what we'd learned about community efforts having greater likelihood of success than efforts grounded in the government sector, and given our evidence-based hypothesis that the unique community social structure in Palau may well be a key pathway for creating positive, sustainable change, we chose to work most closely with Ulkerruil A Klengar (UAK), a community health group serving all of Palau but based in Ngerbeched, and with a track record of creating health-based radio and television programming.

In 2013–2014, funding from the Tanita Healthy Weight Community Trust supported the creation of 20 live radio programs on different nutrition and food production related topics. These programs were hosted by Palauans (with occasional guests from outside of Palau) and were recorded in both audio and video for re-airing. Importantly, Palau's few radio stations, combined with high rates of radio use in Palau, mean that these health messages had strong listenership.

While the radio and television programs were reaching Palauans on a large scale, we focused the bulk of our efforts on adapting the NHLBI's "We Can!" nutrition education program curriculum for use in Palau, including selection of topics that seemed most pertinent given interview findings (information about healthy food selection, encouraging healthier snacks, preparing healthy meals, and coping with busy schedules). The program was originally designed as a series of in-home nutrition demonstrations, but was ultimately implemented by UAK in a series of larger group gatherings across Palau, making particular use of Parent-Teacher Association meetings and school assemblies. UAK's selection of knowledgeable and well-respected Palauan program facilitators (who were not government officials) meant that over 700 Palauans participated in the "We Can! Palau" program in July and August of 2014. Program evaluations reveal great interest in the topics covered and suggest additional topics for future programming. The curriculum remains in the hands of UAK and other Palauan agencies.

The lion's share of the effort described above was targeted to Palauan adults (though several children attended "We Can! Palau" sessions). We also wanted, though, to heed the advice of Palauans such as this respondent: "The best way to encourage Palauans? I think the best way is to start with the kids. I noticed that Palauans now are listening to their kids more often, when you, when the kids come home and they say, oh, yeah mom I learned this that you know, let's just grow our own cabbage, our own eggplant, our own, things that have a big impact." To begin developing effective means of influencing childhood nutrition in Palau we have partnered with Ministry of Education officials, who expressed strong interest in learning more about parent, teacher and student perceptions of nutritional curricula and policies both in the schools and at home. Lancey (this volume) conducted research with parents and teachers at Koror Elementary School in Ngerbeched, finding strong interest in enhanced school-based nutrition programming and policy.

Lancey's work, combined with interview data and positive feedback from the "We Can! Palau" programming in schools, paved the way for May 2015 focus groups with students, parents and teachers in four Palauan elementary schools—including schools in Ngerbeched and Ngarchelong, along with another school in Koror and the school in Peleliu (the third site profiled by Labarthe and colleagues in 1973). We based this phase of our research in part on youth nutrition-based Community-Based Prevention Marketing work conducted in Kentucky (Bryant et al. 2010) and worked with Ministry of Education officials to develop instruments with questions about definitions of healthy and local foods, benefits and barriers associated with consumption of these foods, and insights and ideas about school nutrition curricula and policies. Analysis of the 21 focus groups is ongoing, but preliminary data have been shared with the Ministry of Education and used in training workshops. The coming months and years will bring continued work in development and assessment of curricular and promotional materials and provision of data that might favorably influence school policy relative to nutrition.

"THE PEOPLE WHO HAVE A RIGHT ON IT": CONCLUSION

Sadly, the health indicators that Labarthe and colleagues measured in the early 1970s have changed for the worse in Palau, despite over 40 years of subsequent public health intervention. There are aspects of the applied anthropological endeavor that, we hope, might convert Palauan insights and ideas into positive new directions for change. Of course, as in many global health efforts, when we set out to create a program of applied research in Palau we could not have predicted with certainty the direction of the work, the ideas and insights of the target population, nor the stakeholders who would play key roles. Looking five years out, however, we are able to identify some aspects of the work that have been particularly fruitful. First, from the very earliest discussions in 2010 we planned for our work in Palau to be longitudinal. In hindsight, not only did this demonstrate a level of commitment to Palau that is perhaps novel in a public health infrastructure that is heavily reliant on short term grants and what Costello and Zumla (2000) term "parachute research," but it also freed us to be more reactive to the stated needs of stakeholders and to develop small-scale test programs that yield important lessons for the development of larger efforts. In short, there is no quick fix to Palau's NCD problems, so it seems clear that Palau is best served by long term research and community change strategies.

Second, this project was designed in the best traditions of an applied anthropology that seeks to be as inclusive of stakeholders as possible (Drake 1989). This has been especially crucial in Palau, where the small population magnifies interconnectedness. We've utilized these powerful social networks to establish relationships with government agencies, community agencies, and key community figures, leading to improved questions and improved data collection from significant percentages of target populations in Ngerbeched, Ngarchelong, and now the four 2015 study schools. These partnerships are especially crucial to our plans for ongoing implementation of nutrition programming. For example, if a new school nutrition curriculum has the support of teachers, but not the support of the parents, it is unlikely to be reinforced in the students' homes. The same applies to the teachers. If the curriculum is not favored by those in charge of its delivery, it will not be properly implemented within the school.

Third, while recognizing the clinical realities of NCD, we have seen great benefit in situating our study of Palauan nutrition in more squarely social and global terms. Palauans are far more likely to speak of imported food and Westernized work days when they speak of the nation's NCD issues than they are to speak of calorie counts and fat grams. We see great value in designing public health promotion strategies that connect with local perceptions of the issue being addressed. Finally, we have sought to conceptualize our research in a manner that eschews the sorts of colonial structures that continue to be reified in much contemporary global health. Our work with Palau is not yet another form of international aid, but rather a collaboration wherein we see Palauan ideas as capable of inspiring meaningful change in global nutrition-based NCD rates. In short, in the tradition of applied anthropological practice, we have endeavored to work together in an effort to privilege the voices of "the people who have a right on it."

Chapter 2

Applying a Socio-Ecological Model to Obesity in the Caribbean

A Community-Based Approach at the Tapion Hospital in Castries, Saint Lucia

Colleen O'Brien Cherry and Elizabeth Serieux

Chronic disease is on the rise in middle income countries like Saint Lucia, which are undergoing simultaneous epidemiological and nutritional transitions (Gaziano and Pagidipati 2013). A range of social, cultural, economic and environmental factors have been posited as an explanation for the global increase in chronic diseases and their associated risk factors, yet it is not clear how these factors interact at both the micro and macro levels to influence individual behaviors and population health (Smith et al. 2014). This chapter reports on a qualitative study conducted in Castries, Saint Lucia between 2012 and 2014. The overall objective of the study was to characterize perceptions and beliefs about lifestyle practices that are associated with increased risk for cardiovascular disease (CVD), with a particular focus on obesity and psychosocial stress. Applying an emic perspective to people's perceptions and beliefs about CVD and its associated behaviors can ultimately help to inform public health interventions and make them more appropriate for Saint Lucians who are at risk for CVD. The data are analyzed using a socio-ecological model approach to understand the multi-leveled social, cultural and economic factors that have contributed to the increase in CVD in a local setting in Saint Lucia.

SAINT LUCIA: A MIDDLE INCOME COUNTRY IN TRANSITION

Saint Lucia is a middle income country with a population of approximately 163,362, the majority of which is black (85%), followed by a mix of black and East Indian (11%), East Indian (2.2%) and unspecified/other (1.7%).

English is the official language, but the French patois *Kweyol* is widely spoken, especially among older members of the population. The island is divided into eleven districts, but the most heavily populated area is the capital city of Castries. Castries is located in the north of the island and serves as the business and administrative center as well as being home to 28% of the population. Saint Lucians remain a mostly rural population, but the urban population is growing rapidly due to a growing tourism and services industry primarily in the urban districts of Castries and Gros Islet, both located in the northern part of the island.

Saint Lucia is a country in transition. These transitions often include lifestyle changes, like changes in physical activity and food consumption patterns (Offer, Pechey, and Ulijaszek 2010; Ulijaszek 2007). In the late 1990s, Saint Lucia transitioned from an agricultural to a service sector and tourism based economy. This transition was prompted simultaneously by policy changes that disturbed their foothold in banana exports and by the eradication of diseases like schistosomiasis, an acute and chronic disease caused by parasitic worms, which spurred more foreign visitation to the island (Ellis 2005). However, the new service and manufacturing industry was not able to replace the former income from banana industry (Greaves and Amarelu-Marshall 2010).

The shift from a primarily agricultural-based economy to a service and tourism economy was accompanied by rapid urbanization. Ongoing ethnographic research in the country has revealed the associated changes in living arrangements, family relations, eating habits and general lifestyle (Cherry et al. 2014). The people of working age migrated to cities from the villages and rural areas in search of jobs, leaving behind the young and the old. Although Saint Lucia is a small island, the nature of the work found in the service industry and the road conditions do not lend themselves to daily commutes. Young children left in the villages were now being raised by their grandparents who in turn were burdened by the financial and social responsibilities of raising a second generation of children. In many cases this left women unable to fully support themselves financially and the women were therefore dependent on their children, other relatives, and the government social security system for assistance. The influx of people into the urban areas of the island has resulted in overcrowding and has put additional stress on the social services in Castries and the other larger towns.

As people relocate for jobs they often lose their social support systems. Social marginalization of this kind has been tied to high rates of CVD in the Sami cultural group living in Norway (Bent-Martin Eliassen 2013). Fechner (2011) found a similar pattern of social change in Germany after the collapse of socialism tied to changing cultural processes and an increase in psychosocial stress and illness, particularly where it concerned threats to individual social and economic security. This type of cooperation for collective advancement is giving way to a more individualistic pursuit of success and a more competitive culture in Saint Lucia and participants expressed this as one of the main sources of psychosocial stress in their daily lives.

NON-COMMUNICABLE DISEASES AND CARDIOVASCULAR RISK FACTORS IN SAINT LUCIA

Non-communicable diseases (NCDs) such as type II diabetes and CVD are increasing globally, and there have been astronomical increases in disease prevalence in low- and middle-income countries over the past several decades (WHO 2014). Although chronic diseases like CVD have in the past been primarily associated with wealthier countries, this is no longer the case. The World Health Organization (WHO) reports that chronic diseases are a growing epidemic, responsible for the deaths of approximately 38 million people each year. The vast majority of those deaths (approximately 75%) occur in low- and middle-income countries. In addition to causing death, NCDs also decrease quality of life, they reduce personal and national productivity, and they are expensive to treat at both the personal and national levels. The current high rates of NCDs in these countries, coupled with continued high rates of infectious disease, can also cause the "double burden" of disease. Furthermore, the health systems are often not equipped to deal with the long term care of chronically ill patients. This can lead to premature death and disability due to chronic diseases that are both treatable and preventable, younger populations being affected by the diseases, and sometimes catastrophic health expenses. A growing burden of NCDs can affect national economies via reduced labor, lower productivity and increased health expenditures (Council on Foreign Relations 2014).

Reducing NCDs in low- and middle-income countries requires an understanding of how socio-cultural contexts shape lifestyle choices and behaviors related to modifiable risk factors for CVD. Of particular interest is identifying how individual, community, and global-level factors interact with one another to influence health and well-being. This research was designed to address this need for socio-cultural understanding by using semi-structured interviews and focus groups to elicit cultural beliefs, perceptions, and practices concerning understandings and beliefs about CVD and its primary risk factors.

Saint Lucia's rapid urbanization has prompted a more sedentary lifestyle in line with new employment and greater exposure and access to convenience and fast foods, all of which have contributed to an increase in risk behaviors for NCDs. In Saint Lucia, risk factors for NCDs that are associated with the epidemiologic and economic transitions include obesity, unhealthy diet, sedentism, alcohol consumption, smoking and stress. Obesity, one of the primary risk factors for CVD and other NCDs, is rising worldwide and at an especially fast rate in middle-income countries like Saint Lucia (WHO 2014). Obesity is on the rise throughout the Caribbean where many countries are experiencing economic and health transitions (Rueda-Clausen, Silva, and López-Jaramillo 2008). An estimated 74% of Saint Lucians are overweight or obese (WHO 2011). The causes of obesity are complex and include shifting cultural norms about fat acceptance and body size, increased caloric intake and decreased caloric expenditure, and less nutritional foods (Popkin, Adair, and Ng 2012). Ongoing ethnographic research in Saint Lucia reveals that women tend to accept larger body size than a North American ideal (Cherry et al. 2014). Some of the other behavioral risk factors associated with obesity are food and dietary changes, increased alcohol consumption, sedentism, and chronic stress.

Obesity is an important risk factor that contributes to development of chronic disease, increases the risk for serious health problems, reduces quality of life, and quadruples an individual's risk for premature death (Teague, Mackenzie, and Rosenthal 2013). Obesity may also cause negative social and economic consequences at the individual, family, community and country levels. The harmful effects of obesity are expressed in a variety of ways: some are as direct as the physical stress placed on the body by carrying extra pounds and others are more complex, involving hormonal and metabolic changes (Cherry et al. 2014). The negative health effects of carrying excess weight begin as early as when BMI reaches the level classified as overweight. An excess amount of weight places undue strain on the body's skeletal framework, particularly on the joints. The knees, hips and lower back are particularly susceptible to this strain, causing pain and discomfort even before the onset of clinical disease (Colditz 1992). This pain and discomfort typically limit mobility and since limited mobility reduces physical activity this in turn exacerbates weight gain.

One of the pathways through which obesity leads to disease is the development of metabolic syndrome. Metabolic syndrome refers to a cluster of symptoms that increase a person's risk of development of NCDs (Cherry et al. 2014). A person with metabolic syndrome is twice as likely to develop heart disease and five times more likely to develop diabetes than a person who does not have metabolic syndrome.

Saint Lucia's health system is not equipped to address the magnitude of health problems that the populations currently face. The health system is currently comprised of public financing, private external funding (fees, loans, grants, donations), private insurance, and out of pocket expenses (Johnson and Stoskopf 2010). Saint Lucia operates 33 health clinics across the island where people can go to get subsidized care; mostly acute and some preventive care. However, there are limited resources and long lines at these community clinics. There are currently five hospitals, four public and one private, that offer more specialized services, but these costs are often not all covered under the country or private insurers' health plans. There have been decreasing trends in public spending and the public health budget. Patients seeking care in health facilities often need to pay out of pocket for fees for medical and hospital care, dental and ophthalmological, and laboratory exams. There are also additional required fees for copayments for drugs and hospital stays. Quality along with the cost of health care has been an issue as a result of limited technology, limited funding and an over-taxed system (Johnson and Stoskopf 2010). Johnson and Stoskopf note that screening and treatment for NCDs has been particularly lacking in the Saint Lucia healthcare system.

Lifestyle intervention strategies can be successful at helping to prevent NCDs, but it's important for these interventions to be culturally based to ensure their success. In 2011, colleagues who work as cardiologists at the Tapion Hospital, a private hospital in Castries, Saint Lucia contacted the authors at the Center for Global Health at the University of Georgia with concerns about the growing number of patients they were seeing with risks for CVD and metabolic syndrome. As a result of this request, the authors have been involved since 2011 with collecting data on modifiable risk factors for CVD and metabolic syndrome in Saint Lucia. The results will have direct public health significance to our colleagues at Tapion Hospital who have collaborated with us on the studies and who are using the results to develop health interventions to educate patients and provide preventive care in the clinical setting.

ELICITING SAINT LUCIAN CULTURAL UNDERSTANDING OF CVD AND ITS RISK FACTORS

This research integrates novel methodological approaches from behavioral and health sciences. The study is based on a qualitative design utilizing focus groups and individual interviews to help determine a Saint Lucian cultural understanding of risk factors associated with NCDs. Using focus groups and in-depth interviews to explore the culturally-based beliefs and practices concerning modifiable CVD risk factors provided rich ethnographic data for understanding lifestyle behaviors. Ultimately, an ethnographically grounded approach to disease prevention allows for more population appropriate and successful public health solutions (Smith et al. 2004).

Focus groups are particularly useful for evaluating research sites and study populations, generating hypotheses or propositions, and developing surveys and interview schedules. The photovoice method was used in the focus groups. With photovoice, participants use cameras to take photographs on a specified theme, and then the group reconvenes and the photos are then used as prompts for group discussion. The photovoice method was used as a means to stimulate discussion during the focus groups by providing a visual means of communication between group members and moderators. Photovoice can stimulate reactions and discussions on topics which may be hard for participants to articulate using only verbal communication, such as "What do you think is a healthy body size?" Photovoice has been used extensively in anthropological and public health research and is considered participatory research in that it involves the direct collaboration of participants who are affected by the issue being studied (Hergenrather, Rhodes, and Bardhoshi 2009; Green and O'Neill 2003). Through this process the research participants are able to voice their concerns, understandings, and personal perspectives, to address health concerns and to create collective strategies to overcome them. The method is recognized to be both educational and empowering to study participants (Catalani and Minkler 2009).

Two sets of focus groups were conducted, one with seven participants and the second with five participants. Themes highlighted from interviews in earlier pilot research were used to shape the questions for the focus groups. The focus groups lasted approximately two hours each. Participants were compensated for their time with a monetary incentive ($20) for each focus group that they attended. The emphasis of the focus groups was on the participants' views of heart health, food, nutrition, exercise, lifestyle, stress and social support. After attending the first set of focus groups, the participants were given cameras and were asked to use them in their home and/or community environments to capture the topics discussed in the focus group. Three days later, both groups reconvened. Participants discussed their pictures using the PHOTO discussion questions as a guide (Hergenrather et al. 2009) which required participants to describe their picture, relate what is happening in their picture, explain why they took the picture, describe what this picture tells about their life, and share how this picture provides opportunities to improve their life. The four focus groups dialogues were taped and transcribed verbatim and detailed moderator notes were taken during each focus group by a designated member of the research team. Transcriptions and moderator notes were coding by two members of the research team using NVivo software to identify and organize themes and participants quotes related to obesity and diet change.

In-depth ethnographic semi-structured one-on-one interviews were conducted with 25 people who visited the Tapion Hospital in the capital city of Castries, Saint Lucia. Purposive convenience sampling has been successfully used by researchers to conduct research on cultural models or norms in various settings. The method of employing a convenience sample of visitors to

Tapion Hospital was used during our prior pilot research resulting in a cross-section of the population from nine island districts with an age range of 17 to 96. The sample size of 25 selected for the interviews is typical when conducting in-depth ethnographic interviews that will result in a large amount of text data. Interview questions were constructed based on the literature on CVD risk factors in Caribbean populations, pilot study results (Cherry et al. 2014), and relevant literature on CVD risk factors and obesity studies. Interviews lasted between 30 minutes to 1 hour and participants were compensated for their time with a monetary incentive ($20). Each interview was taped, verbatim transcribed, and coded by two members of the research team. Initial code list selection was conducted independently by the two authors, with cross-checking and final selection done corroboratively until one code list was created. Data were analyzed using NVivo software to identify and organize codes related to a number of domains including: diet, obesity, tobacco use, alcohol consumption, body size, and exercise.

A social ecological model approach was used to understand the social, economic, and political factors that have contributed to the increase in obesity in Saint Lucia (Bronfenbrenner 1977). The social ecological model is a set of interlocking circles that represent different levels such as individual, interpersonal, institutions and organizations, community and societal structures, policies and systems (see Figure 2.1). In its application here, it represents a micro and macro view of factors involved with CVD risk factors. This model has been applied to health behavior broadly and specifically to obesity prevention and program design in various settings (McLeroy et al. 1988). McLeroy et al. note that this model divides the social environment into analytical *levels* in order to examine patterns of behavior in individuals and groups. Individual factors include personal modifiable behaviors such as food intake and exercise, personal beliefs, and biological characteristics. The interpersonal level involves family, friends and social networks. The organizational level involves institutions such as schools, religious institutions and the workplace. The community level involves the neighborhood environment including greenspaces and access to physical activity, types of food stores, fast food outlets, and restaurants. Finally, the public policy level represents local, state, and global structures including the media, agricultural policies, food production and distribution systems, government and public policy and societal norms and stigmas about obesity.

When an individual decides upon a particular course of action, like whether or not to engage in a health behavior, s/he takes all of those other factors into consideration. Individual behaviors are influenced and conversely limited by the contexts within which they find themselves (Kahn, Yang, and Kahn 2010). Consequently, it is imperative that health beliefs and behaviors also be viewed and addressed within this framework. The

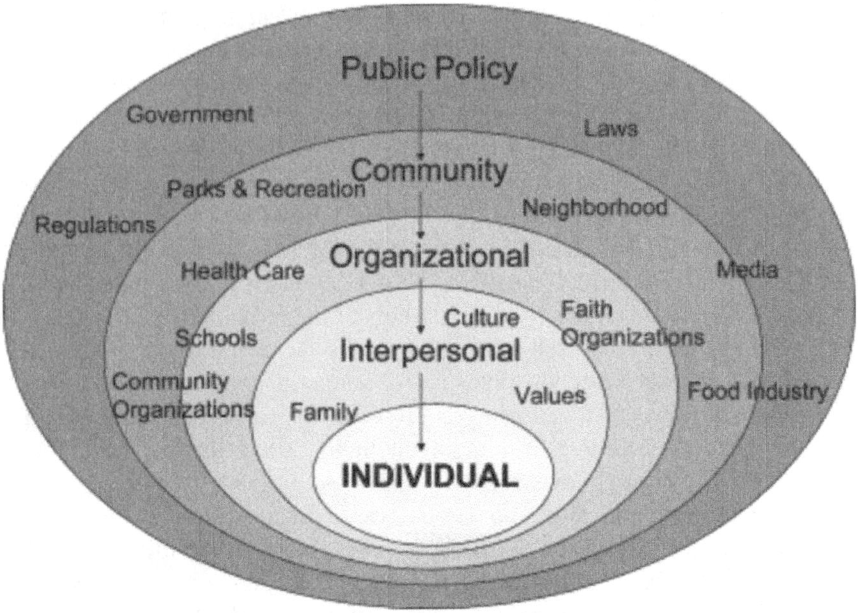

Figure 2.1 Social Ecological Model

social ecological model includes where people live, play, work, eat, shop, exercise, the factors that influence these decisions and the impact that their subsequent actions have on diet. The model illustrates the wider global context and the impact that it has on the island of Saint Lucia and then in turn there is a depiction of the environment in Saint Lucia and how that affects the possibilities and options that are available to the Saint Lucians as they navigate through life.

DIET AS A PRIMARY RISK FACTOR FOR CARDIOVASCULAR DISEASE IN SAINT LUCIA

Study participants identified diet as the most important risk factor for CVD. They also identified it as the easiest factor to change. Interviews and focus groups reveal that participants have a substantive knowledge of how to eat "healthy" for heart health. The foods they named that are healthy foods include both local and imported fruits like mangoes, bananas and apples as well as vegetables like pumpkin, tomatoes, and root vegetables like dasheene. Typical Saint Lucian food is described as healthy overall but high in carbohydrates. One participant said, "A Saint Lucian plate of food includes meat, ground provisions, plantain, green figs, yam, dasheene, sweet potato and then you get rice or you get pasta." This statement was made in support of the perspective that not only are the typical Saint Lucian foods high in carbohydrates, but a wide variety of these foods are eaten during meals; further increasing the carbohydrate consumption and also contributing to large portion sizes, which are also typical in Saint Lucia.

The transitions that are taking place in Saint Lucia have also changed food preferences and introduced new foods at the individual, interpersonal, and community levels. Fast foods and convenience foods are considered more modern than traditional foods and are perceived to fit better with a fast-paced urban lifestyle. One participant commented that consumption of fast foods is now more common especially in the urban younger generations, "young people are eating all these fast foods you hear the statistics and stuff and a lot of them they go to work, they don't cook at home they eat fast food and a lot of them find themselves having heart attacks and all these other diseases." The high availability of inexpensive, calorically dense but nutritionally poor food has altered the general nutritional environment so although large amounts of calories are being consumed the nutritional value of those calories is very low. The relatively inexpensive costs of some high caloric foods has influenced consumer buying behavior. For example, one participant described her decision to take advantage of a two for one deal on pizza, "So we bought two because there was this promo, buy one large pizza and get the other one free at Dominos. So we took full advantage of that. We were stuffing our faces with as much as we could get . . . so we definitely would not have decided to get a pizza, but since there was a deal we decided to use it."

Foods that were once traditional and more commonly available and eaten are now more expensive than some imported foods or processed convenience foods. One participant commented, "Food on the whole, vegetables everything, have gotten expensive, right now a banana is $.25 sometimes $.50, well it depends on the size but yes it's gotten really expensive."

Participants discussed diet change over the past couple of decades at length and emphasized how the diet of their grandparents in particular was different from their own diet. There was general consensus among the participants that some of the more recently adopted foods like pasta that are commonly eaten today as staples and as special "Sunday foods" during family gatherings were not eaten by older generations. One participant said, "My grandmother would never eat macaroni and cheese" which is a dish now commonly served on Sundays when friends and family gather to eat and socialize. Older generations also reportedly ate less meat and when they did eat meat, it was leaner then than it is today. A participant indicated, "Another thing too that the meat they used to eat probably was only on special occasions if you looked at some of the pork and the beef we have now . . . the fat that is in there, because they're fattening these animals up for us, they didn't have that, their meat, their animals were leaner and it was eaten healthier."

The overall perception as stated by participants is that it is more challenging today in Saint Lucia to eat healthily than it was in the past. Furthermore, participants emphasized that costs of traditional foods such as fish, fruits and vegetables are rising dramatically. They attributed the rise in food prices in part to the recent government implementation of a 15% value added tax (VAT) implemented in 2013. Several participants stated: "Eating healthy in Saint Lucia is very expensive." The net effect of this situation is that although people are aware of the foods that are healthy and those that are not, often times, they have to choose between healthy food and food that they can afford. One participant said,

> I will go to the store and be like radishes yes, yes I should eat that. But then I look at the price and turn around and go find something less expensive because most persons on the island, a majority of the population is made up of middle class people and low socio-economic people where you have electricity bill, water bill and all of these things increasing and with the advent of VAT, it makes it more difficult to eat what you know you are supposed to for the sake of your health, because it is costly. So, instead of eating a bowl of salad and having to buy more vegetables on a weekly basis, you eat a lot more breadfruit, more than one slice, because that is what is falling off the tree at the back of your house.

Foods that participants deemed healthy like fish, fruits and vegetables were described by several as "expensive" and a "delicacy" due to their high prices. One participant said, "They [children] like fruit but it is expensive—you give a child a slice of pineapple and it's like one of their favorites you know it's gourmet, even ripe bananas have gotten expensive." The current price of bananas was discussed at length and was viewed by participants as one of the more direct examples of the rising costs of food at the public policy level. In earlier times when Saint Lucia's economy was primarily agriculturally-based and bananas were the main export crop, surpluses of this fruit were very common and bananas could be obtained for very little and sometimes for free. This case with bananas was used by participants as the prime example to support their perception of how rapidly things have changed with regard to the availability and price of foods that are perceived as healthy in Saint Lucia.

Participants indicated that one of the main effects of this change is that they have to budget and plan in advance if they want to consume healthier alternatives. One participant described her efforts to eat healthy as often as her budget allows:

> When I shop I interchange so I say okay I'll buy fish so that's all I'm eating this month and next month I'll do chicken because I can't do fish in two months consecutively because it's too expensive (group yes) and you buy a tray of fish with probably like three steaks of fish and it's almost 30 dollars do you know how much chicken that can buy?

Another, somewhat overlooked consequence of the rapid change from eating local, unprocessed foods that were primarily obtained from family and friends to eating processed foods primarily obtained from a supermarket shelf is that the importance of reading food labels is neither fully appreciated nor widely practiced. The foods grown on someone's farm or in the backyard do not have labels, neither does the fresh catch of fish at the docks, therefore, the necessity of reading labels is a fairly new phenomenon, and is generally not practiced to the necessary extent. Some participants indicated that even in the cases when labels are read, they remain unsure of what exactly they are looking for. Therefore, according to participants, the decision to purchase and consume food becomes even more financially based than nutrition related, since people do not read labels because they are unaccustomed to it or because the tools to distinguish the "healthier" unhealthy options from the marginally more healthy ones are non-existent.

Along with changes in health behaviors at the individual level, the participants also reported changes at the interpersonal level (between and among individuals). One of the biggest changes at the interpersonal level seems to be a shift from a more collective culture with strong family ties, close kinship networks, and a more informal economy for food (and other goods and services) to a more individualistic society with looser social connections and more incorporated into a globalized economy. At the individual level, residents have often lost ties with family and other close social networks as they've moved to cities to find new opportunities in the growing tourism economy. Losing these close ties has reportedly caused stress for many participants in this study and has diminished the use of an informal economy by which to obtain local foods. On the other hand, it has become more expensive to participate in the formal economy and purchase healthy options. Therefore, at the individual level, participation in Saint Lucia's informal economy as a method of obtaining food has become more difficult and has diminished, while participation in the more formal economy is generally restricted to purchasing the less expensive options, many of which are calorically dense but nutritionally empty.

An example of the shift from the use of informal economy and a more collective, cooperative culture to a more formal, individually based culture is the dying tradition of the *koudemain* (Saint Lucian kweyol) from the French *coup de main*, which means "to lend a hand." A *koudemain* is what occurred when individuals wanted to accomplish an activity that they could not do by themselves, examples would be clearing a piece of land, building a wall or a house extension. The individual would supply all of the building materials as well as food and drink for the day, while family, friends and community members would come together and supply all of the necessary labor. According to one of the participants, the shift away from a cooperative culture has resulted in higher levels of stress as individuals feel more socially isolated, and adds to the growing culture of competitiveness and individualism.

There have also been significant changes at the policy level in Saint Lucia. The most significant of those changes is the recent implementation of the VAT. This policy change has influenced spending behavior at the individual level, since it has made eating healthy in Saint Lucia more expensive. Another consequence is that it has decreased the amount of disposable income available to most Saint Lucians and therefore they have reduced "non-essential" purchases like gym memberships, further reducing the likelihood of participation in other healthy, stress reducing activities.

Much like the situation with the bananas, participants agreed that there has been a rapid and drastic change in both the availability and price of fresh fish. Once plentiful and inexpensively purchased, this has also become prohibitively expensive. The participants explained that the high cost of fish is due to the high price of fuel to take the boats out to where the fish are, and the fact that there are fewer fishermen. Therefore, the combination of fewer fishermen faced with rising costs of plying their trade, results in fewer fish, which are in turn sold more expensively to the general public.

Additionally, globalization of food at the policy level has influenced food preference and availability at the individual and community levels. The food industry has introduced new products, many of which are processed and high in sugars, fats and carbs. The major threats to health from these processed foods have been shown to come from sugar sweetened beverages as well as high levels of fat and sugar that are added to foods to increase their palatability (Margaret 2011). These are some of the main ingredients in the foods that have become increasingly common on the island, and since both novelty and palatability influence the amount of food that is eaten, the convergence of these factors in the food supply has contributed to the increase in obesity in Saint Lucia. Offer and colleagues have referred to this phenomenon as "food shock," describing ever cheaper and more accessible foods that have been linked with obesity in their research on affluent countries with market-liberal welfare regimes (Offer, Pechey, and Ulijaszek 2010). Further, at the interpersonal level the values assigned to food are changing and factors like convenience, taste and modernity have become more important. Interestingly, anthropological food studies often highlight the strong cultural connections of eating practices and foods to nostalgia and to cultural norms. Food habits are often the hardest and the last things to change during periods of cultural transition (Kittler and Sucher 2011). Additionally, breaking out of established patterns of cultural eating practice is difficult and often overrides latent concerns about health and wellness (Wilson 2010).

CHRONIC PSYCHOSOCIAL STRESS AS A SECONDARY RISK FACTOR FOR CARDIOVASCULAR DISEASE IN SAINT LUCIA

Economic vulnerability creates a stressful environment where individuals are forced to rapidly adapt and transition to new jobs, lifestyles and neighborhoods often leaving behind a strong social network when they relocate to urban areas. Participants recognized and stated that stress is bad for heart health, that built up stress can cause a big stomach, and that stress may cause other health problems. They cited some of the primary causes of stress in Saint Lucia as money, family, social competition, and general lifestyle issues. Stress has prompted changes in multiple areas of the socio-ecological model, including individual, interpersonal, and community levels. Many individuals in our studies described living in Saint Lucia as stressful. Individuals who are experiencing psychosocial stress may turn to various coping methods including dietary behaviors which place them at higher risk for CVD such as eating of high caloric "comfort" foods or binge drinking of alcoholic beverages.

Referencing the interpersonal level, several of the participants stated, "People stress about money." This is described as a cultural change in spending habits and debt obligations. One participant said, "People have taken on more debt in Saint Lucia and this has caused stress and suicides because they can't pay their bills." Others referred to less tangible social sources of stress stating, "It's hard to rise up and improve yourself. Others want to keep you down with them." Several participants described Saint Lucians as being competitive with one another and so striving for success causes stress as others whether directly or indirectly try to thwart your efforts. During focus group discussion, participants talked about how this competition can be seen in the consumptive practices of Saint Lucians to buy Western goods such as expensive clothing or cars that may signal their "success" to others.

Family life is also viewed as a source of stress. Caring for children both financially and otherwise causes stress and families often fight over money. Much of the stress is attributed to economic pressures from the new VAT tax, the bad economy, and high rate of unemployment. Additionally, participants indicated that even among those who are employed, the shift away from traditional agriculture (which typically took place in farms close to home, around the island) to a more centralized service sector has caused people to move away from the traditional central family home and rent or buy a house closer to the new place of employment and thus incur more living expenses.

In addition to increased expenses, those people who move away from their families and communities for employment opportunities find themselves in unfamiliar living conditions with little or no social support available to them. Participants indicated that typically individuals who move closer to their place of employment return "home" as often as they can, sometimes every weekend. Therefore, they do not typically have the chance to form new relationships in their "home away from home." This adds to the burden of stress that is attributed to many of the lifestyle realities of living in urban Saint Lucia. Participants stated that in addition to stress caused by the new social realities, just living in the city is itself a stressor. They cited traffic and driving as causes of stress, and they also indicated that the inherent busyness of the city and a lack of time cause stress. Several participants discussed the perspective that although there are so many different factors that contribute to the high levels of stress experienced, there is not much known about effective methods of handling or coping with stress. As a result, many people attempt to dissipate stress in counterproductive ways including overeating, smoking and drinking alcohol. All of these behaviors are risk factors for non-communicable disease.

The overall result of these social, cultural, economic and policy changes has reportedly been an increase in stress which in turn has changed people's health behaviors with over eating and overconsumption of alcohol perceived as ways to "cope" with the stressful environment. Stress affects all levels of the model, from the individual trying to survive on their own in a rapidly changing immediate environment, to the pressures that have resulted in less social support systems to the national policy environment as the country's leadership struggles to find and implement methods to generate revenue and make Saint Lucia competitive in the global environment.

CONCLUSION

Taking a socio-ecological model approach to analyzing local data about obesity and health highlights micro and macro level connections and interactions that do not appear linked on the surface. Research results indicate that people understand that food that is closer to its natural state as being healthier than the more processed versions. However, their decisions regarding which foods they will actually consume are based on interlocking economic, social and cultural factors. The end result is health behavior that places the population at risk of obesity and associated non-communicable diseases. Effective interventions at the local level should take into account that factors influencing behavior span more than one level of the model and therefore all domains should be addressed and be included as important considerations when planning and implementing public health strategies.

BEST PRACTICES

Based on the results of our research in St. Lucia, we have learned the following lessons that should be applied to planning and implementing future CVD prevention programs:

- Many efforts to understand NCDs and associated risk factors do not take a cultural or community-based approach and have subsequently been unsuccessful. Lifestyle intervention strategies can be successful at helping to prevent CVD in at-risk populations, but it is crucial for these interventions to be culturally based.
- The importance of using qualitative research methods to understand and characterize the drivers of behavior is often overlooked. However, (and particularly in behavioral sciences) the information that can be obtained from using qualitative methodology is a perfect complement to that obtained by using other more quantitative means and is central to designing behavior change interventions.
- Research results should be used to create cultural and community-based lifestyle intervention strategies and educational materials that incorporate local understandings, language and concerns.
- Obesity is a complex risk factor with many different socio-cultural, economic and political causes. Obtaining local level perspectives that pertain to the social ecological model can help practitioners determine how the different levels (individual, interpersonal, organizational, community and policy) affect each other, and this information can be used to inform policy change and program implementation to mitigate negative effects of the policy changes at the community and national levels. It may highlight areas of most concern such as economic or environmental factors where resources could be pooled.

Chapter 3

Anthropology Field School Insights into Community-Based Participatory Research to Address Food Insecurity[1]

The Case of Demonstration Keyhole Gardens in the Monteverde Zone, Costa Rica

Lillie Uyên-Loan Đào, Sara Arias-Steele, Emily Bissett, Constanza Carney, and Zuhra Malik

In 2013, the Globalization and Community Health (GCH) interdisciplinary field school was in its first year of a three-year National Science Foundation funded grant that combines the applications of anthropological and environmental engineering theories and methods to address community health issues in the Monteverde Zone (MVZ) and San Luis. The GCH field school is an intensive nine-week summer program conducted in the MVZ in association with the Monteverde Institute and the University of South Florida. With its focus on a cross-disciplinary perspective, the field school provides students with hands-on, rigorous training on methods from anthropology and environmental engineering to conduct community health research in the MVZ. During the field school, students are given the opportunity to engage in rapid ethnographic assessment by working with local health-related institutions (i.e. hospitals, clinics, and health centers), farmers, grassroots organizations, community-based organizations, and government agencies as well as with personnel from the Ministry of Health, the School of Public Health at the University of Costa Rica, and with community organizers.

For this exploratory study, the 2013 cohort of the GCH field school investigated intergenerational perspectives on local agricultural practices, issues of food access, and perceived benefits and barriers to personal gardening with the goal of addressing food insecurity in the MVZ. Located in the province of Puntarenas in Costa Rica, the MVZ includes the towns of Monteverde, Cerro Plano, and Santa Elena. The 2013 cohort also collaborated with residents of the neighboring town of San Luis for this study (see Figure 3.1). Framed by a

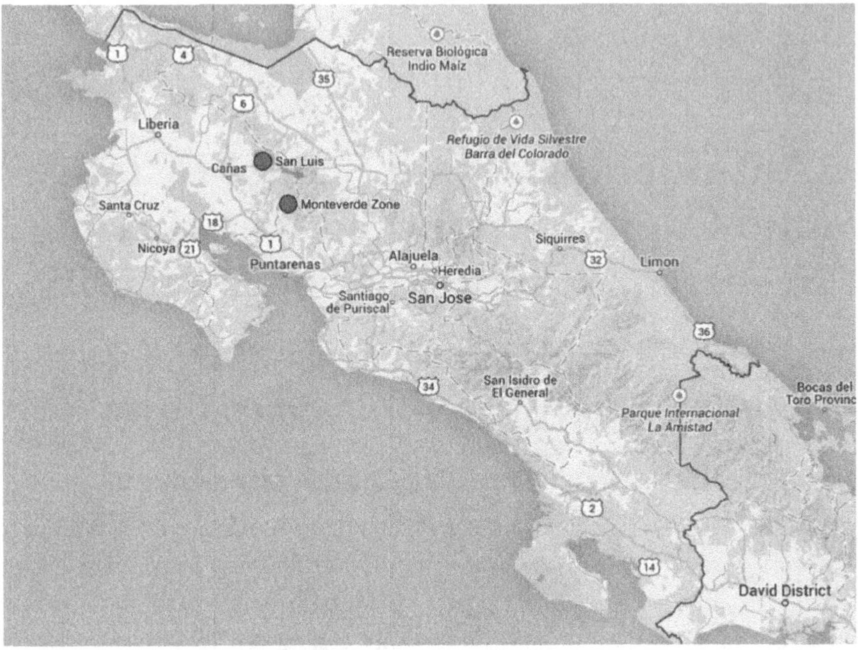

Figure 3.1 A map showing the location of the Monteverde Zone and neighboring town of San Luis, indicated by the circles (created using Google Maps, 2015).

critical pedagogical framework (Freire 2000), community-based participatory research (CBPR) was employed to gather qualitative and quantitative data by drawing from rapid ethnographic methods. While conducting CBPR to gain local understandings of values and practices related to food insecurity in the MVZ and San Luis, gardening emerged as a potential facilitator to mitigating local food security as it was identified by local residents to increase access to reliable, fresh, and organic produce. Subsequently, researchers undertook the project of adapting a Keyhole gardening method to the region in pursuit of working with the local communities to reintroduce agricultural practices as a means to addressing the adverse effects of food security.

ECOTOURISM, FOOD DELOCALIZATION, AND LOCAL FOOD INSECURITY

Due to a coalescing of several sociopolitical factors, the rural communities in the MVZ are transitioning from an agriculturally-centered to ecotourism-based economy. Agriculture has traditionally been the main source of income and sustenance for residents of the MVZ, but in recent years an increasingly competitive global food market combined with the rise of the ecotourism industry has led to the decrease in community-driven food production. As with many agriculturally-rich countries competing in the global market, Costa Rica has shifted their land use[2] for the purposes of producing cash crops (i.e. cocoa, coffee, tobacco, and sugar cane) rather than growing produce for local consumption. This has largely attributed to the price inflation of locally available foods, pushing families in lower-income communities to adapt to an ecotourism-based economy as a means of sustenance. Additionally, Costa Rican environmental policy-makers have strengthened their commitment to preserving their country's natural resources and to sustain its biodiversity in the past decade. Not surprisingly, at the same time, ecotourism began to see a significant rise in popularity. In particular, ecotourism takes center stage in the MVZ's local economy as it is home to the famous Monteverde Cloud Forest Preserve, the Children's Eternal Rainforest, and the Santa Elena Rainforest Preserve. Accordingly, MVZ has experienced heavy traffic by researchers, tourists, and organizations interested in the conservation of natural environments and improving the welfare of local people and cultures. While there have been identifiable benefits of the rising ecotourism industry,[3] a continuously increasing exposure to tourists has also served to further aggravate the region's growing community health issues. Previous research done in the MVZ revealed that a significant number of families who were involved in tourism exhibited some degree of food insecurity (Himmelgreen et al. 2006, 2013).

Data from past research on the state of community health in the MVZ established that food insecurity is a rising concern for residents as reflected in the high rates of obesity and cardiovascular disease resulting from a diet comprised of mostly processed fast foods rather than home-cooked meals (Himmelgreen et al. 2006, 2013). Moreover, measuring food insecurity using the Radimer/Cornell[4] scale, previous research also indicates that more than half of the Monteverde households that were sampled (n = 193) exhibit some form of food insecurity, with 68.39% of those households involved in the tourism industry. Past research in the MVZ posits that there is an important relationship between the recent economic shift, food insecurity, and health outcomes experienced by community MVZ members (Cantor et al. 2013; Himmelgreen et al. 2013; Rhee et al. 2012; Himmelgreen et al. 2006; Whiteford 1992).

Food insecurity in the region has transitioned from food scarcity (i.e. limited food availability) to food inadequacy (i.e. limited variety and lower nutritional quality) (Cantor et al. 2013; Himmelgreen et al. 2013; Himmelgreen et al. 2006). Local food insecurity is shown to be exacerbated by (1) the consumption of high amounts of fast foods or frozen processed meals due to convenience, (2) long working hours not allowing time to cook meals at home, and (3) the high cost of local produce (Himmelgreen 2006). MVZ residents have highlighted that a disproportionately high amount of people who work in the local ecotourism industry often feel as though they lack the time required to prepare meals, thus altering their nutritional choices (Allen 2012). As a result, food insecurity in this region is characterized not necessarily by decreased food quantity, but by decreased access to a variety of quality food items (Himmelgreen et al. 2006; Simon 2014). These patterns manifest themselves in rising rates of obesity and overweight— factors that increase the risk for chronic health problems such as hypertension, diabetes, and cardiovascular disease (Martin and Ferris 2007; Himmelgreen et al. 2006).

As the local realities of a competitive global food market persist and the ecotourism industry continues to thrive in the MVZ and its neighboring regions, the communities' means for sustenance have moved away from localized food production and towards an increased reliance on the ecotourism industry. Parallel to this, participation in family gardens or small farms, an activity that could alleviate the effects food insecurity, has declined at the local level. Researchers engaged with the MVZ and San Luis communities to explore the relationship between food insecurity and agriculture. This chapter will discuss how the researchers implemented CBPR and critical pedagogy in exploring local agricultural practices and the community values that surround it. This chapter will then discuss the resulting implementation of a demonstration Keyhole garden.

COMMUNITY-BASED PARTICIPATORY RESEARCH AND CRITICAL PEDAGOGY

Researchers employed the tenets of critical pedagogy—a transformative approach to education—to frame CBPR in order to address issues associated with local food insecurity. CBPR is research that is done *with* and *for* a community and not merely *on* or *in*. This form of research is a partnership of students, faculty, and community members who collaboratively engage in research with the purpose of affecting social change (Strand 2003; Freire 2000). The egalitarian foundation of CBPR provides all parties involved with an avenue for empowerment to work towards civic engagement in the evolving project of democracy. CBPR promotes a form of research that not only includes participatory and action-oriented methods, but also advocates for education to be utilized as a tool to encourage transformative social justice. Leaders in CBPR (Strand et al. 2003) equate critical pedagogical CBPR with the democratization of knowledge in which (1) knowledge brought to the project by all partners involved is equally valued; (2) multiple research methods are used; (3) accessible and appropriate approaches to the dissemination of knowledge are provided; (4) and, in accordance with critical pedagogy's dialectical nature, conventional assumptions about knowledge itself are challenged. The research team implemented a CBPR framed by critical pedagogy with a broader goal of promoting the transformative model of education as opposed to the one that acquiesces to the status quo.

METHODS

In their collaborative approach to addressing local food insecurity, researchers with the GCH field school integrated the following methods through a critical pedagogical CBPR approach: participant observation, free listing, pile sorting, focus groups, open-ended interviews, structured interviews, and grounded theory analyses. This exploratory study combined both qualitative and quantitative methods in order to obtain cross-disciplinary understandings of the investigated variables. The methods implemented in this investigation are based on the operationalization of the following variables: (1) generational knowledge of agriculture, (2) produce access and attainment, (3) current gardening practices, and (4) the level of interest in gardening.

As part of the participant observation efforts, all six researchers resided in home-stays with local MVZ and San Luis families and were actively involved in the Monteverde Institute's day-to-day events and activities that engaged with local residents. Additional rapid ethnographic assessments included free lists and pile sorts (n = 12) that were administered one-on-one with MVZ and San Luis participants. Participants were asked to free list the reasons why they would want a personal garden. Participants were then asked to rank the listed reasons on a scale of one to four on their level of importance. Following the free list and pile sort activities, two focus groups were conducted: the first in San Luis (n = 6) and the second in the MVZ (n = 8). Open-ended interviews (n = 4) were then administered to individuals who work in farming and agriculture in the MVZ and San Luis. Oral questionnaires (n = 61) were conducted at the 2013 San Luis Educational and Recreational Fair, at supermarkets, and farmers markets located in both the MVZ and San Luis. Utilizing an interview schedule, participants were asked to respond to as nearly identical a set of stimuli as possible. Recruitment of participants for this study was made possible by the Monteverde Institute and the University of South Florida staff and faculty's already established rapport with MVZ and San Luis community leaders and gatekeepers who led the recruitment process.

Grounded-theory analyses were implemented to record and manage the qualitative textual data sets that included field notes and transcriptions of interviews, focus group discussions, and open-ended responses derived from the oral questionnaire. Grounded-theory is a set of systematic techniques for discovering patterns in human experiences that utilizes close, inductive examination of unique cases combined with the application of deductive reasoning. The aim is to discover theories—causal explanations involving the investigated variables—grounded in empirical data (Bernard 2011, Strauss et al. 1994). The grounded-theory method relies on coding texts for themes, then analyzing the themes for data. Quantitative data were also derived from analyzing survey responses using SPSS Statistical Analysis and Software.

EXPLORING LOCAL AGRICULTURAL KNOWLEDGE AND PRACTICES

CBPR was conducted through a partnership between MVZ and San Luis communities, the Monteverde Institute, the University of South Florida, and the 2013 GCH field school cohort. This CBPR was aimed at exploring the relationship between food insecurity and local gardening knowledge and practices. MVZ and San Luis community members exhibited significant interests in personal gardening, particularly in creating a demonstration gardening project to advocate for the increase of local agriculture practices. Themes that emerged from rapid ethnographic assessment of reasons for obtaining a personal garden included: (1) increased food access, (2) improved produce quality, (3) the promotion of intergenerational communications on local agriculture, and (4) decreased food delocalization and ultimately a buffer to the negative effects of food insecurity currently experienced by families in the MVZ and San Luis.

Local Agriculture Emerges as Facilitator to Address the Adverse Effects of Food Insecurity

The mitigation of food insecurity and produce delocalization are themes that were derived from qualitative inquiry into the benefits of local agriculture and gardening. Increased food quality and improved food access were most frequently identified by free list and pile sort participants as reasons for obtaining a personal garden (see Figure 3.2). Moreover, conversations with MVZ and San Luis community members during open-ended interviews, focus groups, and oral questionnaires further reinforced increased food quality and

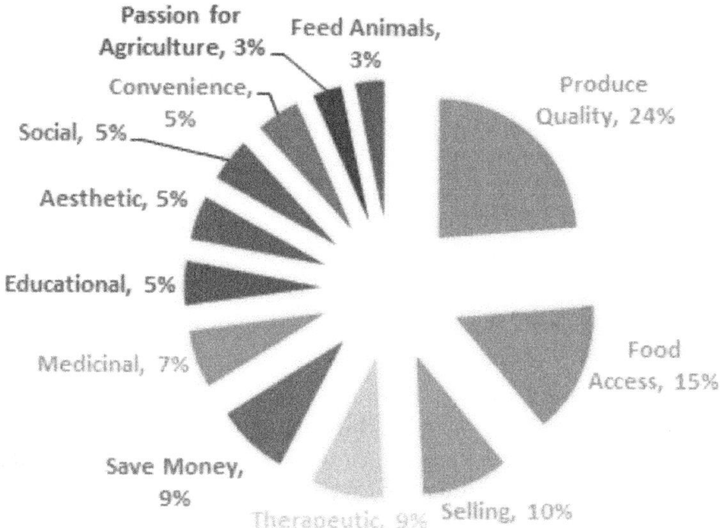

Figure 3.2 Frequency of cited reasons to have a personal garden identified by MVZ and San Luis participants during free list and pile sort activities (n = 12).

access as significant and critical reasons for obtaining a personal garden. During rapid ethnographic assessments, questions and discussion topics that were posed included the following: (1) What are the benefits and advantages of engaging in local agricultural practices? (2) What are the challenges and disadvantages of engaging in local agricultural practices? (3) What role has agriculture played in your life? (See Figure 3.3). In response to the posed questions and topics, an interview participant stated that a benefit of having a garden is "to have produce without chemicals and free of preservatives" (June 25, 2013). Similarly, a focus group participant discussed the adverse effects of the use of chemicals and added that, "In the market, we don't know what we're eating [referencing the previous discussion on herbicides]. When you grow your own food, you know what you're eating" (June 27, 2013). A prominent theme, the desire for quality produce was also discussed by another participant when he discussed his wish for organic fruit stating, "For me who likes to cook, sometimes I go to the market and I find that the tomatoes look orange, it looks like they used a lot of chemicals. I don't like that." (July 17, 2013). When asked about agriculture and its benefits, challenges, and role in personal wellbeing, a vast majority of the participants emphasized the importance of organic cultivation and the nutritional benefit of retaining agriculture within the community.

Examples of questions and discussion topics posed during rapid ethnographic assessments with Monteverde Zone and San Luis community members

- What role has agriculture played in your life?
- Degree of prevalence on local agricultural knowledge in the community
- Values tied to traditional local agricultural practices
- What are the benefits and advantages of engaging in local agricultural practices?
- Ideas for the promotion of the benefits agricultural practices
- What are the challenges of engaging in local agricultural practices?
- Ideas for resolving the challenges of agricultural practices
- What are the effects of food insecurity in your community?
- Ideas to address local food insecurity
- Introduction of the Keyhole gardening method
- Feedback on the idea of creating a demonstration Keyhole garden locally
- Feedback on how to adapt the Keyhole gardening method locally
- Potential advantages and disadvantages of a local Keyhole garden

Figure 3.3 Examples of questions and discussion topics that were posed during the following rapid ethnographic methods administered with Monteverde Zone and San Luis participants: in-depth interviews, focus groups, open-ended oral questionnaires, and surveys.

The vast majority of MVZ and San Luis participants identify local agricultural knowledge and practices as deeply beneficial to community health and family livelihoods. During initial discussions on local agricultural practices and the values that surround these practices, community members expressed a heightened concern about a decline in said practices. Focus group and open-ended interview participants associated the decline in local agriculture with a gap in generational communication.

The Generational Gap in Valuing Local Agriculture

Previous research done with the MVZ and San Luis communities revealed that participation in family gardens or small farms, an activity that could buffer against food insecurity, has declined at the local level (Himmelgreen et al. 2006). Specifically with younger generations, this pattern is seen in their shift from pursuing agriculture-related careers to pursuing jobs in the tourism industry. This shift has led to a generation gap in the knowledge on local agricultural production and its benefits to community health. During focus groups, older parents and grandparents in the MVZ and San Luis expressed their concern for the loss of agricultural knowledge in their younger generations. During these conversations, elders made their sentiments clear by urging that a continual decrease in local agricultural practices and knowledge will lead to detrimental effects on their health and livelihoods. Furthermore, elders went on to discuss potential ways to fill this generational gap on agricultural knowledge. Several community members cited gardening as a promising means for the facilitation of agricultural knowledge and practices between generations. Despite this gap, when researchers posed questions about the idea of implementing a demonstration small-scale garden—specifically, a Keyhole garden—participants of all generations indicated that personal gardens may not only bridge the generational gap, but also serve to provide families with improved food quality and access, ultimately buffering local food insecurity.

Subsequent to qualitative inquiry about local agricultural practices and the values that surround these practices, we administered oral questionnaires at the 2013 San Luis Educational and Recreational Fair where MVZ and San Luis residents were in attendance. Oral questionnaires included both open-ended questions and survey-like questions regarding feedback on and levels of interest in the implementation of a demonstration Keyhole garden. When asked how interested one would be in constructing a demonstration community Keyhole garden, most participants (82.14%) indicated that they were either interested or very interested. Similarly, the vast majority of the participants (89.29%) stated that they were interested or very interested in constructing a home Keyhole garden. In accordance with critical pedagogical CBPR done with the MVZ and San Luis community, researchers undertook the project of implementing two demonstration Keyhole gardens on the Monteverde Institute grounds located in the MVZ.

INTRODUCING THE KEYHOLE GARDEN TO THE MONTEVERDE ZONE

What is a Keyhole Garden?

The Keyhole garden is a compact permaculture technology originally implemented in sub-Saharan Africa to increase access to fresh produce in vulnerable populations (Mathule 2009; McCarthy 2004; Romero-Daza et al. 2009). Keyhole gardens contain a basket in the center for organic kitchen waste to feed plants and replenish the soil's nutrients (Keyhole Garden Manual 2009). The combination of the center basket and the angular entranceway gives the garden a Keyhole shape when viewed from above, increasing accessibility and limiting pests (see Figure 3.4). The garden uses a number of layers to nourish the soil, proven to catalyze production. The garden is constructed from low-cost, recycled, reusable and local materials

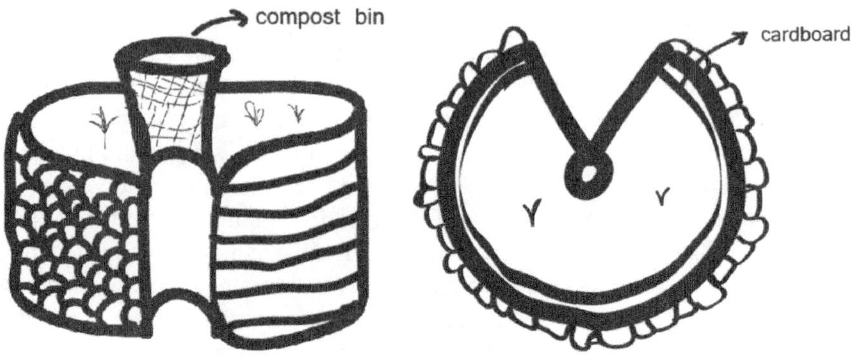

Figure 3.4 Front (left image) and overhead (right image) views of a basic keyhole garden model.

and is two meters in diameter and one meter in height. While the compact Keyhole garden has been successfully used to increase access in food insecure communities living in dry climates, this exploratory study marks the first attempt to implement this particular type of gardening method in a wet and windy climate.

Local Insights on the Keyhole Garden

Focus groups and oral questionnaires administered with participants at the local farmers market, supermarkets, and during the Educational and Recreational Fair provided community members with the opportunity to share perceived benefits, disadvantages, and personal impediments to the construction of a Keyhole garden. Focus group discussions revealed that the three greatest potential benefits are the Keyhole garden's environmentally friendly features, its functional structure, and its promotion of self-sufficiency. The fourth most frequently cited potential benefit is the Keyhole garden's associations with healthiness. Participants discussed its health benefits in the context of overall wellness to encompass physical, mental, emotional, and social health. An interview participant described the potential therapeutic benefits of a personal Keyhole garden referring to her son who has engaged in personal gardening to aid in his successful battle with substance abuse (see Figure 3.5).

While CBPR and rapid ethnographic assessments confirm that the vast majority of participants cite more benefits than disadvantages, participants also expressed a few challenges pertaining to certain Keyhole garden features. They provided feedback and suggestions for improvements during focus groups and open-ended interviews. The majority of the perceived disadvantages were derived from questions regarding the structural integrity

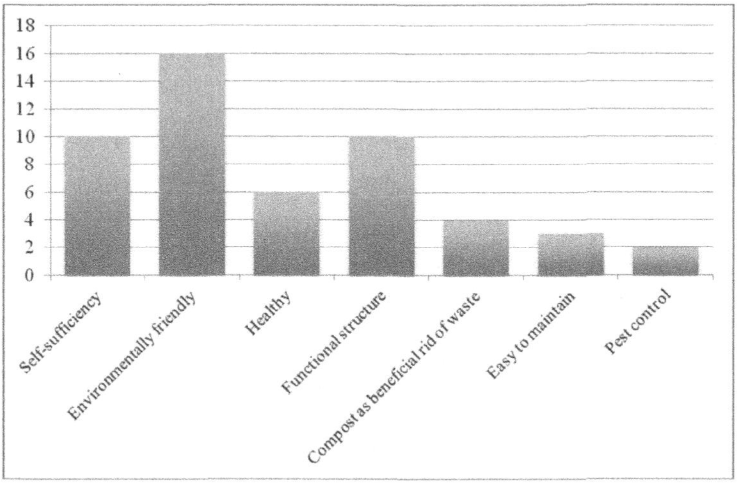

Figure 3.5 Frequency of potential Keyhole garden benefits identified by MVZ and San Luis participants during focus groups and questionnaires (n = 61). The Y-axis indicates the number of individuals that cited the particular benefit.

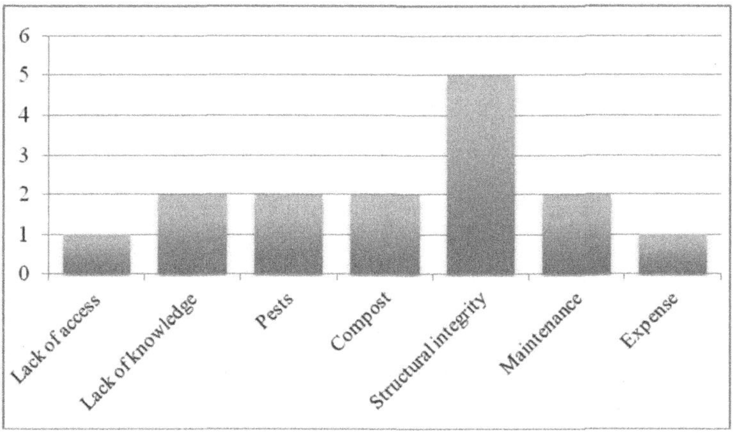

Figure 3.6 Frequency of potential Keyhole garden challenges identified by MVZ and San Luis participants during focus groups and open-ended interviews (n = 18). The Y-axis indicates the number of individuals that cited the particular challenge.

of the Keyhole garden against environmental factors specific to MVZ and San Luis. Community input also revealed additional concerns related to the compost pests, general maintenance, and a current lack of knowledge on how to build the specific Keyhole garden. General maintenance apprehensions centered on questions of time and required upkeep needs such as weeding and watering the garden (see Figure 3.6).

The extreme environmental features of the MVZ combined with the presence of a long tradition of agriculture made these findings fairly expected. In response to community feedback on the original Keyhole garden method, researchers proceeded to inquire with great breadth and depth on ways to properly modify the original Keyhole garden method to fit the context of the MVZ.

Adapting the Keyhole Garden Method to the Monteverde Zone's Context

Previous research in the MVZ highlights the prominent agricultural tradition present in the MVZ and San Luis communities (Himmelgreen 2006). Open-ended interviews with agricultural experts aimed to understand these traditions in order to develop a community and climate appropriate adaptation of the Keyhole garden. MVZ and San Luis residents discussed both traditional and new gardening practices with the 2013 cohort during interviews and focus groups. Themes included pest control methods, composting processes commonly practiced in the region, and cultivation strategies for rain and wind.

The topography of Monteverde presents various individual microclimates fluctuating between periods of heavy rain, high winds, and dense humidity, with annual rainfall averages of 118 inches (3,000 mm). Humidity oscillates between 74% and 97% (Nadkarni 2000). Interview and focus group participants referenced these extreme climate conditions in the context of feedback on the necessity to implementing a roofing system. Based on participant feedback, the 2013 cohort designed roofing systems made of both the saran and a greenhouse clear plastic for the two demonstration Keyhole gardens.

The significant amount of rainfall in the MVZ factored largely into the local adaptation of the Keyhole garden. In the original design of the Keyhole garden, water filtration and drainage was not a factor due to the arid climate of sub-Saharan Africa. However, the MVZ poses the opposite problem with an intense rainy season. Based on community input from MVZ and San Luis participants, two differing drainage mechanisms made using locally sourced, sustainable, and readily available construction materials. One drain was constructed by reusing glass bottles while the second drain was made of stacked, large stones. In the months after the completion of the two demonstration Keyhole gardens, plant growth and water filtration aided in determining which drainage system functions most adequately.

Surveys and focus groups revealed a wide variation of compost ingredients available, such as manure (i.e. chicken, cow, horse, goat, and rabbit), carbon material (i.e. leaves, dry trunks, "gransa de arroz" or the outer covering of rice grains), and differing material to maintain a neutral pH in the soil (i.e. limestone, ash, or sawdust). The compost materials that were used for the adapted Keyhole garden were isolated into chicken wire barrels to allow for aeration and then mixed with additional soil and dry leaves for two weeks. This mixture was then mixed with soil and applied to the final layer of the Keyhole gardens.

In order to determine the plants that would be both feasible to cultivate and greatly utilized by the local community, the 2013 cohort asked participants to name the top ten plants that local participants would choose to grow in a home garden. Responses collected from the San Luis Educational and Recreational Fair indicated that the following plants were most frequently desired for cultivation. Starting with the most frequently cited produce desired for cultivation, participants chose: (1) lettuce, (2) tomato, (3) cilantro, (4) sweet chili, (5) cabbage, (6) beans, (7) corn, (8) orange, (9) yucca, and (10) ayote (see Figure 3.7). Based on these research results, selected seeds were organized in the garden to highlight permaculture practices of companion planting and the method of alternating root and shoot vegetables to maximize productivity (Keyhole Garden Manual 2009).

The researchers' use of CBPR in working with MVZ and San Luis communities to investigate potential benefits of the Keyhole gardening method indicated that the reintroduction of local agriculture is a possible means for alleviating food insecurity and addressing concerns about obesity and overweight. Framed by a critical pedagogical approach, the 2013 cohort conducted CBPR with and engaged local residents in dialogues about the issues associated with food insecurity, local agriculture, and the sociopolitical and cultural context of the MVZ and San Luis.

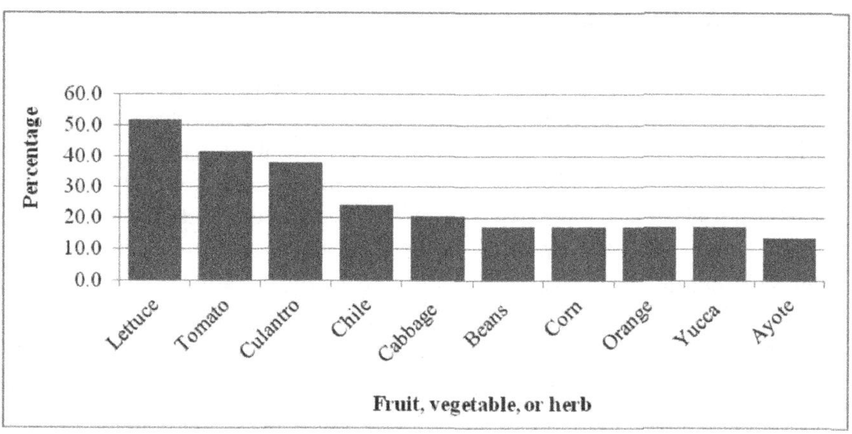

Figure 3.7 Top ten products desired to cultivate as determined by individuals at San Luis Educational and Recreational Fair (n = 31).

INSIGHTS GAINED FROM COMMUNITY-BASED PARTICIPATORY RESEARCH AND CRITICAL PEDAGOGY

The structure of GCH interdisciplinary field school is representative of a transformative model of education that urged all parties involved in the research (i.e. local MVZ and San Luis residents, Monteverde Institute and University of South Florida staff and faculty, and the 2013 cohort) to engage with each other in a critical manner to not only understand, but also to question circumstances surrounding their local and global economies, politics, and culture. It is these kinds of action-oriented understandings that will permit the augmentation of the unfinished project of democracy and make it better suited to the changing conditions of society (Giroux 2011).

In the case of CBPR in the MVZ and San Luis, all parties involved were encouraged to question the current sociopolitical factors that have led to the MVZ's transition from an agriculturally-centered to ecotourism-based economy and subsequent food delocalization. In successfully doing so, a locally adapted demonstration Keyhole garden emerged as a promising facilitator to buffer the adverse effects food insecurity has on community health. The case of the demonstration Keyhole gardens in the MVZ reinforces the efficacy of CBPR as framed by the tenets of a critical pedagogy.

Critical pedagogy[5] frameworks aim to alter the status quo and advocate for social justice. In opposition with the tenets of critical pedagogy is the dominant banking model of education. The banking model of education maintains that students are largely a passive repository of information in which knowledge is deposited by the teacher (Freire 2000). The banking model of education is characterized by a hierarchical dualism manifested in the student-teacher relationship. "Education either functions as an instrument which is used to facilitate integration of the younger generation into the logic of the present system and bring about conformity or it becomes the practice of freedom, the means by which men and women deal critically and creatively with reality and discover how to participate in the transformation of their world" (Freire 2000, 34). Future efforts aimed at working with food insecure communities would benefit greatly by applying the critical pedagogical CBPR approach. This approach promotes an environment that urges civil society to enter critically and innovatively into dialogues about issues facing vulnerable populations to offer potentially transformative solutions.

Framed by these tenets, the CBPR[6] that researchers undertook centered on ways to engage in these kinds of dialogues with local residents to provide potential means for alleviating the disproportionate food insecurity being experienced by families in the MVZ. Dialogue was facilitated by rapid ethnographic assessment in the form of participant observation, free listing, pile sorting, focus groups, and open-ended interviews. These forms of qualitative inquiry provided avenues for critical pedagogical education resulting in insights to inform future efforts in promoting small-scale gardening practices to address food insecurity.

RECOMMENDATIONS FOR FUTURE EFFORTS TO ADDRESS FOOD INSECURITY WITH GARDENING

Critical pedagogical CBPR methods were implemented to engage in dialogues about the facilitators, barriers, and values associated with local agricultural practices, and to also adapt the demonstration Keyhole garden to the culture and climate of MVZ. This exploratory study exhibited the utility of investigating small-scale gardening as a means for local agricultural knowledge and value sharing between generations. Keyhole gardens may offer a space in which traditional and new practices can merge for the benefit of the community. Further research geared towards investigating the relationship between (1) the decline in agricultural knowledge among younger generations and (2) the effects of small-scale gardening on community health, may aid in the deconstruction of generational gap, potentially shedding light on ways to leverage community specific practices toward improved nutritional outcomes.

This CBPR underscores the need to conduct research on the potential for small-scale gardening to improve not only immediate, but also long-term food security. The previously discussed adaptations made to the original Keyhole garden methods provide a base for further research into the effectiveness of the Keyhole gardening methods, their structure and level of productivity. The demonstration Keyhole gardens built at the Monteverde Institute will be monitored by Monteverde Institute staff in the coming years in order to determine functionality, community interest, and future steps. MVI and San Luis residents have expressed interest in the utilization of the gardens for the engagement of local community members in educational programming in this newly adapting gardening method. To aid these efforts, a manual for the construction and maintenance of the adapted Keyhole garden has been developed and distributed to interested community members and potential future partners.

Applications of a critical pedagogical CBPR for the GCH field school work led to a two-fold outcome: (1) a field school experience that successfully permitted the convergence of knowledge, power, and action, creating a transformative model of education for all of parties involved and (2) insights to inform future efforts in promoting gardening practices to address food insecurity and related adverse effects on community health. The case of the demonstration community Keyhole gardens in the MVZ of Costa Rica illustrates how a critical pedagogical CBPR approach is successfully implemented to investigate contextually-sound means to address the adverse effects of food insecurity. As sociopolitical environments continue to shift and exacerbate both food delocalization and food insecurity, the need to explore culturally appropriate and community specific ways to mitigate negative effects on community health become increasingly critical.

NOTES

1. Thank you to the following people who have played critical roles in making this community work possible:

- The community members in the Monteverde Zone and San Luis who have collaborated with us for this community-based participatory research
- All the staff of the Monteverde Institute: Jenny Peña, Gaudy Picado, Toni Salazar Mora, and Randy Picado
- Our community advisor, Milto Brenes
- Alejandro Garcia
- Rigoberto Mendez
- Patricia Jimenez
- Those who helped us with constructing the demonstration Keyhole gardens: Aaron Hockman, Mario Cordero Badilla, Golberto Cordero Badilla, and Giraldo Algedas
- Our professors: Dr. David Himmelgreen, Dr. Nancy Romero-Daza, and Dr. Sarina Ergas
- Our Graduate Assistants: Allison Cantor, Stephanie Paredes, and Adib Amini
- The National Science Foundation: "REU Site Globalization and Community Health: Combining Social Science and Engineering" Grant No. 1156735 (PI, Nancy Romero-Daza, Co-PI David Himmelgreen)

2. For further reading on the relationship between local agricultural production, the global market economy, and land use, refer to Eric F. Lambin and Patrick Meyfroidt's article "Global land use change, economic globalization, and the looming land scarcity" (2011).

3. For further reading on ecotourism in Costa Rica, refer to Elizabeth Boo's book "Ecotourism: the potentials and pitfalls: country case studies" (1990).

4. For details on measures used in the Radimer/Cornell, refer to Anne Kendall, Christine M. Olson, and Edward A. Frongillo Jr.'s article "Validation of the Radimer/Cornell measures of hunger and food insecurity" (1995).

5. For in-depth reading on the critical pedagogical framework of this research, refer to Paulo Freire's book "Pedagogy of the Oppressed" (1968), particularly his perspective on the banking model of education.

6. For further reading on applications of community-based participatory research done in the context of community health, refer to Meredith Minkler and Nina Wallerstein's book "Community-based participatory research for health: From process to outcomes" (2011).

Chapter 4

Community Approaches to Obesity Prevention in Brazil

The Food and Nutritional Security Paradigm

Charles Klein

In the past 15 years, Brazil has made food and nutritional security a centerpiece of national social policy through its *Fome Zero* (Zero Hunger) initiative. Originally proposed in 2001 by Worker Party's presidential candidate Luiz Inácio Lula de Silva, the program became a reality with Lula's election as President of Brazil in 2002. Zero Hunger starts with the premise that achieving food and nutritional security in Brazil requires an explicit shift in Brazil politics and economic policy.

The right to quality food is an inalienable right of all citizens, and it is the State's duty to create appropriate conditions for the Brazilian population to enjoy this right. The audience to be contemplated in this proposal is large—9.3 million very poor families (or 44 million people) earning less than a dollar a day. There is hunger in Brazil not for lack of food, but for lack of money in the pockets of workers to buy it (Silva 2001).

Seeking to address poverty-related food insecurity, in 2005 the Lula administration launched *Bolsa Família* (Family Allowance), a conditional cash transfer program that provides an average monthly stipend of approximately R$70 (about US$34 using the average currency exchange rate over the past five years) to very low income families (incomes below US$56) in exchange for proof that their children are vaccinated and attending school (Soares, Ribas, and Osário 2010). In its first ten years, the Bolsa Família program reached over 11 million families for a total of 50 million individuals (Ministério de Desenvolvimento Social e Combate à Fome [MDS] 2012, World Bank 2015). Research suggests that most of the Family Allowance has been spent on food consumption (Duarte, Sampaio, and Sampaio 2009; Mourão and Macedo 2012). In combination with economic growth, rising wages and old age pension expansion, the Family Allowance has helped lift an estimated 20 million people out of poverty in the past decade (Kilpatrick

2011; Neri 2010, 2014). This poverty alleviation has greatly reduced food insecurity in Brazil and enabled the country to reach two benchmark hunger policy objectives: (1) the Millennium Development Goal 1 (MDG-1) target of halving the proportion of hungry people by 2015, and (2) the 1996 World Food Summit (WFS) target of halving the absolute number of hungry people by 2015 (FAO 2014a, b).

Despite these impressive advances in reducing hunger, Brazil's food and nutritional policymakers face a second challenge—rapidly rising obesity rates. According to a national survey commissioned by Brazil's Ministry of Health in 2012, 51% of adult Brazilians are overweight (up from 43% in 2006 and 19% in 1975), and 17% of adults are obese (up from 11% in 2006 and 3% in 1975) (Government of Brazil 2013). As in other middle-income countries experiencing nutrition transitions (Foster et al. 2014; Kandala and Stranges 2014; Popkin, Adair and Ng 2012; Zhang et al. 2012), the increase in the number of overweight Brazilians is linked to changing food practices and more sedentary lifestyles (Conde and Montero 2014; CONSEA 2010). This nutrition transition is demonstrated by declines in the consumption of fruits and vegetables (in 2002/2003 only 23% of the population met WHO's recommendation of five or more portions per day); decreases in the consumption of traditional Brazilian foods such as beans, rice and cassava or manioc; and increases in the consumption of saturated fats, processed foods and soft drinks, (CONSEA 2010; on the spread of Big Food in Brazil, see Monteiro and Cannon 2012; on Big Food globally, see Williams and Nestle 2015).

In this chapter I explore how Brazil has responded to obesity prevention through the development of an intersectoral food and nutritional security paradigm (*Segurança Alimentar e Nutricional*/SAN) rather than the medicalized disease/epidemic framework that dominates obesity discourse and policy in many wealthy nations, including the U.S. The Brazilian food and nutritional security framework was consolidated into law in 2006 with the enactment of the *Lei Orgânico de Segurança Alimentar e Nutricional* (LOSAN-Lei ° 11.346/Food and Nutritional Security Law), which established the *Sistema Nacional de Segurança Alimentar e Nutricional* (SISAN/National Food and Nutritional Security System) (Leão and Maluf 2012). Key institutional components of this multilevel system include:

1. The *Conferência Nacional de Segurança Alimentar e Nutricional* (National Conference on Food and Nutritional Security), at which representatives of civil society (two-thirds of participants) and the government (one-third of participants) from all of Brazil's 27 states come together every four years to debate and set food and nutritional security policy priorities;
2. The *Conselhos de Segurança Alimentar e Nutricional* (Food and Nutritional Security Councils), participatory governance bodies at federal, state and

municipal levels that propose priorities, recommendations and budget levels and provide advice on state-directed food and nutritional security policies;
3. The *Câmara Interministerial de Segurança Alimentar e Nutricional* (CAISAN/Interministerial Chamber for Food and Nutritional Security), which, based on the recommendations of the National Conferences and the national CONSEA, develops, monitors and evaluates food and nutritional security policies and the four-year national food and nutritional security plans; and
4. The amendment of the Brazilian Constitution to include the *Direto Humano Alimentação Adequada* (DHAA/Human Right to Adequate Food) (CONSEA 2010).

In applying this still evolving food and nutritional security framework to obesity prevention activities, Brazilian policymakers have concentrated on the cultural, economic and political factors affecting healthy eating (CAISAN 2011; Conde and Monteiro 2014). This emphasis on the structural determinants of healthy eating and obesity is clearly articulated in the final proceedings of the 2007 III National Conference on Food and Nutritional Security, the first national food and nutritional security conference at which obesity issues received significant attention (Government of Brazil 2007, 19–20). The discussion begins with a statistical description of the increasing numbers of overweight and obese Brazilians across all social strata. The text then outlines the complex causality behind these developments, including "an increase in the consumption of high fat and sugar foods, urbanization, an increase in industrialized foods, the automation of everyday activities, an increase in motorized transportation, and a reduction of physical activities." The document notes that these changes in food culture (e.g., more eating out and more processed foods) and food systems (e.g., expanded agricultural output generating low priced, industrialized foods of poor nutritional quality) have supported a disproportionate rise in obesity in populations with lower income and education levels. In conclusion, the text connects these national processes to international "free market" (quotes in original) economic forces that support unhealthy eating (e.g., industrialized agriculture, Big Food) and that work against governmental and international efforts to promote food and nutritional security.

Four years later, obesity issues moved to center stage on the food and nutritional security policy agenda when "Reversing Obesity" was named a priority on the first page of approved proposals at the IV National Food and Nutritional Security Conference ("Adequate and Healthy Food: Everyone's Right") (Government of Brazil 2011, 32–33). The Reversing Obesity proposal states that

> Public policy should articulate through the entire food system, from production until consumption, guaranteeing food that meets the principles of variety,

> quality, balance, moderation, pleasure and taste; gender, race and ethnic dimensions; cultural and regional specificities; and environmentally sustainable product that values organic agriculture and agroecology, free of physical, chemical and biological contaminants and genetically modified organisms. (Government of Brazil 2011, 33)

Building on these recommendations, the 2012–2015 National Food and Nutritional Plan identifies "Reversing the Tendency for Rising Rates of Excess Weight and Obesity" as the third of the plan´s ten enumerated challenges, and the documents lists specific obesity and excess weight reduction priority goals for children, adolescents and adults (CAISAN 2011). The 2015 National Plan also requested the development of an Intersectoral Obesity Prevention and Control Plan, which the federal government released in January 2014 (CAISAN 2014). This plan calls for the creation of an Intersectoral Management Committee to coordinate obesity prevention and control activities and identifies six primary axes for action:

> (1) Availability and access to appropriate food, (2) actions of education, communication and information, (3) promotion of healthy lifestyles in specific environments, (4) food and nutritional surveillance, (5) comprehensive health care of the individual with overweight/obesity in the health system and (6) regulation and control of the quality and safety of food. (CAISAN 2014, 15)

The remainder of this chapter focuses on on-the-ground examples of the food and nutritional security paradigm in action. I begin with an overview of several national and regional programs that explicitly seek to transform the structural landscape of food production, distribution and consumption. I then present a case study of the state of São Paulo's *Bom Prato* (Good Meal) restaurant network based on ethnographic fieldwork in the city of São Paulo in July–August 2014. These "Working People's Restaurants" provide low cost, nutritionally balanced meals in aesthetically pleasing, communal settings and provide an innovative model for bridging food security and healthy eating. I conclude by highlighting some of the opportunities and challenges of addressing obesity prevention through a rights-based, food and nutritional security paradigm given the realities of entrenched industrialized food systems.

THE FOOD AND NUTRITIONAL SECURITY PARADIGM IN ACTION

Building on the institutional framework discussed above, in the past decade the Brazilian federal government has implemented a wide array of policies and programs that seek to create more equitable and healthy food systems in the face of the growing hegemony of industrialized agriculture and Big Food (CONSEA 2010; CAISAN 2011, 2014; Conde and Monteiro 2014). Recognizing the financial difficulties experienced by many family farmers, the federal government provides price supports through a *Política de Garantia de Preços Mínimos* (PGPM/Minimum Price Guarantee Policy), and the *Programa Nacional de Fortalecimento de Agricultura Familiar* (PRONAF/National Family Agriculture Support Program) provides credit and training to family farmers. Since the mid-1990s, PRONAF has expanded from 184,000 contracts in 1995/1996 to 1.4M contracts in 2008/2009, and $16B in loans to small-scale producers in 2010/2011 (CAISAN 2011). The federal government, in turn, directly purchases and redistributes family farm production to individuals experiencing food insecurity through the *Programa Nacional de Alimentação Escolar* (PNAE/National School Food Program), the *Programa de Aquisição de Alimentos* (PAA/Food Acquisition Program), and the *Programa de Alimentação de Trabalhador* (PAT/Worker Food Program). These policies help small-scale farmers generate income while simultaneously developing efficient systems for distributing healthy foods to lower-income Brazilians, such as the 45M students and 13M workers reached in 2010 through the National School Food Program and the Worker's Food Program respectively. Through offering affordable and convenient options to fast food, these programs seek not only to reduce food insecurity, but also to help stem the rising obesity rates associated with the ongoing Brazilian nutritional transition.

Complementing state-directed structural interventions are innovative initiatives from the private sector, such as *Cozinha Brasil* (Brazilian Kitchen). This cooking and nutrition training program is run by SESI (*Serviço Social da Indústria*/Social Services for Industry), a national foundation supported through contributions from large Brazilian corporations. SESI launched *Cozinha Brasil* on a nationwide basis in 2004 in partnership with the federal *Ministério do Desenvolvimento e Combate à Fome* (Ministry for Social Development and Hunger Reduction), the administrative home of the Zero Hunger program. Brazilian Kitchen offers free 10-hour basic cooking and nutrition courses and a 20-hour professionalization workshop for private sector workers and their families. Over 90% of the students are wives of male workers (Confederação Nacional da Indústria 2008). The program explicitly links good nutrition to citizenship and social inclusion (the program's subtitle is "a recipe for citizenship"), promotes efficient household economics and "smart food" (most of the recipes use low-cost ingredients and cooking by-products that are normally discarded, such as fruit and vegetable peels), and explicitly affirms each state's regional cooking cultures. By 2008, over 360,000 students in nearly 1,000 municipalities had participated in the courses (Confederação Nacional da Indústria 2008).

Another prominent actor seeking to transform Brazilian food systems is a growing cooperative agriculture movement, as evidenced by the 1,500 cooperatives and 1M producers represented through the *Organização de Cooperativos Brasileiros* (Andrade and Alves 2013, Brazilian Cooperatives Organization) (Sistema OCB 2013). Many smaller-scale family farmers are also associated with the more politicized *União Nacional das Cooperativas de Agricultura Familiar e Economia Solidária* (National Union of Family and Solidarity Economy Cooperatives) (UNICAFES 2015). An example of such politically engaged, small-scale family farmers is the *Rede Xique Xique de Commercializão Solidária* (Xique Xique Network for Solidarity Commerce) in the northeastern state of Rio Grande do Norte. Founded in 1999, the Xique Xique Network has several thousand members based out of 50 local groups in 12 cities (Dantos 2005; Rede Xique Xique 2015) (Figure 4.1). Reflecting the large numbers of women involved in small-scale agricultural production in Brazil (Butto, Dantas and Hora, 2012), Xique Xique is composed primarily of female farmers. Its logo, the Xique Xique cactus, expresses these women's perseverance and adaptability in the face of the challenging ecological conditions of the drought ridden northeast of Brazil and a social structure long characterized by patriarchy (Santos, 2014). The Xique Xique Network conducts trainings; sells products in farmers markets, operates a store in Mossoró, the state's second largest city; and participates in feminist and solidarity economics networks.

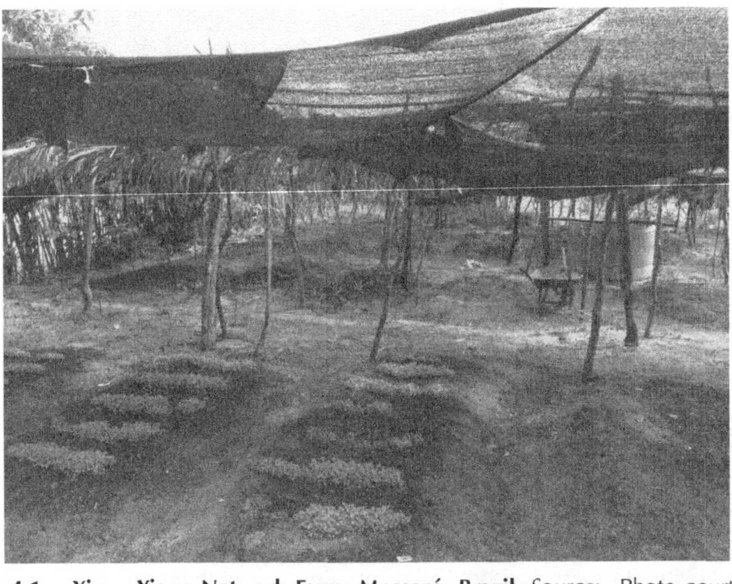

Figure 4.1 Xique Xique Network Farm, Mossoró, Brazil. *Source*: Photo courtesy of Charles Klein.

Through integrating production, distribution and political action, cooperatives such as Xique Xique explicitly seek to offer a model for creating a sustainable and economically just alterative food system that supports income generation, food and nutritional security, and traditional Brazilian food cultures. However, it is important to note that while many Brazilian food and nutritional security initiatives such as Cozinha Brasil and the Bom Prato restaurant network share, at least on paper, Xique Xique's commitment to integrating small-scale producers, regional food cultures, and community building, most are not self-conscious actors in an alternative, solidary economy-based food system. This potential tension between the transformative political rhetoric of food and nutritional policy documents and the on-the-ground realities of developing viable programs in a country with entrenched industrialized food systems is a theme that I will return to in the concluding Lessons Learned section.

BOM PRATO: SUPPORTING HEALTHY EATING

The State of São Paulo launched its *Bom Prato* (Good Meal/Good Dish) Restaurant Network in 2000 with a clear goal: to provide healthy, quality and affordable meals to lower income individuals, the elderly and persons in social vulnerability (Gobato, Pangassi and Villaba 2010). Today, 47 Bom Prato restaurants serve over 80,000 meals per day, and the program has served more than 127M meals through a state government investment of over R$298M (US$145) since its inception (State of São Paulo 2015). Bom Prato is the largest network within a growing movement of nearly 100 *restaurantes populares* ("working people´s restaurants") throughout Brazil. These eateries are typically structured on a multilevel public-NGO partnership model—state or municipal governments cover the majority of operating costs; community-based organizations manage everyday operations, and the federal government finances infrastructure development and capacity building through its Food Access Program and Food Equipment Network programs (MDS 2004, 2015). In July–August 2014 I conducted ethnographic research at the Bom Prato network in the city of São Paulo to (1) examine how state-level bureaucrats and restaurant managers, and customers understand and operationalize the food and nutritional and security paradigm; (2) generate a preliminary profile of Bom Prato customers; and (3) see how Bom Prato affects customer's food consumption and conceptions of healthy eating.

Bom Prato's leadership team explicitly situates their program within Brazil's food and nutritional security paradigm, as was explained to me during an August 2014 interview with the program director, coordinator and nutritionist at the *Secretaria de Desenvolvimento Social* (Social Development

Secretariat), which administers the Bom Prato program for the entire state of São Paulo: "Bom Prato is a state action for nutritional security that supports the fight against poverty and hunger and follows federal guidelines to promote healthy eating. . . . [It is] a vehicle for exercising citizenship" (Bom Prato Nutritionist, August 2014 Interview). In terms of obesity prevention, Bom Prato focuses on "eating well, eating healthy and making good choices" (Bom Prato Nutritionist, August 2014 Interview).

> Obesity is complicated because you can look at a person and say 'ah, that person is overweight.' But you don't know if she is malnourished. You can be overweight and malnourished. . . . In Bom Prato, diners can eat beans, vegetables and fruits everyday. The meal is high in calories – about 1,200 for lunch. But it is balanced in terms of vitamins, minerals, protein, carbohydrates and fats, especially since many individuals only eat this one meal each day. They do not run the risk of obesity by eating at Bom Prato. (Bom Prato Nutritionist, August 2014 Interview)

This nutrition philosophy is aligned with the 2014 national Brazilian food guide, which no longer recommends specific daily caloric consumption and instead emphasizes positive eating practices (Ministério de Saúde 2014).

As of August 2014, the Bom Prato program has formal partnerships with 43 community-based organizations in the State of São Paulo, including faith-based social service organizations, higher educational institutions, and non-faith based, non-governmental organizations. After entering into a contract, the state government provides the managing organization R$400,000 [US$ 194,287] in start-up funds for construction and equipment purchases. On-going operating expenses come from restaurant revenues (R$1.00 [US$ .49] for each lunch and R$0.50 [US$ .24]) for each breakfast served) and state subsidies (R$3.50 [US$ 1.70] for each lunch and R$0.80 [US$ .39] for each breakfast served) (State of São Paulo 2015). In cities other than São Paulo, municipal governments provide an additional R$1 for lunch served. These financial resources support each restaurant's paid staff—a manager, an onsite nutritionist, and 15–20 employees who serve the meals and maintain the restaurant's physical structure. In many restaurants, the managing NGO, which typically does not have experience or expertise in large-scale food service provision, enters into a contract with a third-party contractor who is responsible for sourcing, preparing and serving the food.

The State of São Paulo requires all Bom Prato restaurants to follow nutritional and culinary guidelines set by the program's nutritionist and operationalized by each restaurant's onsite nutritionist. Lunch (*almoço*), the main meal in Brazil, is a complete, 1,200-calorie plate consisting of beans, rice, an animal-based protein, vegetables, salad, manioc flour (a condiment), bread, seasonal fruit, and a beverage. Building on weekly menus developed by the program nutritionist (one dish is offered each day), the restaurants feature traditional Brazilian foods, including the national dish of *feijoada* (black bean stew) on Wednesdays and the regular use of tripe. Diners have the option of choosing two portion sizes, with the smaller portion indicated by the use of a beige tray (Ministério de Saúde 2014). In 2011, the network also began offering a 400-calorie breakfast of coffee, milk or chocolate milk, bread with butter, cheese or cold cuts, and seasonal fruits. The restaurants are open Monday through Friday and serve approximately 300 breakfasts and 800–2,400 lunches per day depending on each restaurant's seating capacity.

In early July 2014, I met with the Bom Prato program staff and arranged for two days of site visits to six restaurants in São Paulo's *Zona Sul* (southern zone). Based on these visits, I selected one restaurant for a more in-depth, ethnographic case study of Bom Prato in action. Like many Bom Pratos, the case study restaurant is located in the so-called periphery, the vast lower-income neighborhoods that surround the more affluent central districts of São Paulo and other Brazilian cities. The restaurant is easily accessed by public transportation—many bus lines pass by the restaurant, and it is a short walk from a metro station. During July and August, I visited the case study Bom Prato approximately twice per week for the entire lunch service, interviewed the restaurant manager and administrative assistant, and, on three separate days in late August, spoke to diners as they were leaving the restaurant after eating. These conversations with diners lasted about two to three minutes and focused on the following topics: (1) how long have you been coming to Bom Prato, and how often do you eat at Bom Prato, (2) what do you think of the food, (3) what do you think of the ambience and clientele, (4) what do you eat at home, and (5) what would you change about Bom Prato. In total, I talked to 51 diners (about half women and half men, with an age range from 18 to 80). Nearly all lived in nearby neighborhoods, about three-quarters had eaten at another Bom Prato, and nearly all lunched every week at this particular Bom Prato, with about half eating there every day.

The restaurant is managed by a nearby faith-based, social service organization, with food services provided through a third party subcontractor. The decor follows the standard Bom Prato layout and aesthetic template (Figure 4.2)—white paint with bright orange accents, light colored tiles, sinks for hand-washing after the payment window and before the food service line, and a large seating area from which diners can view the open kitchen. A medium-sized Bom Prato, the case study restaurant seats approximately 175 people in a cafeteria-style arrangement of 22, eight-person rectangular tables. On a typical day, customers begin lining up for lunch 10–15 minutes before the official 11:00 a.m. opening. At 11:10, the restaurant is half full, with a preponderance of older diners. By 11:30, the restaurant is nearly full and the line extends across the parking area to the sidewalk

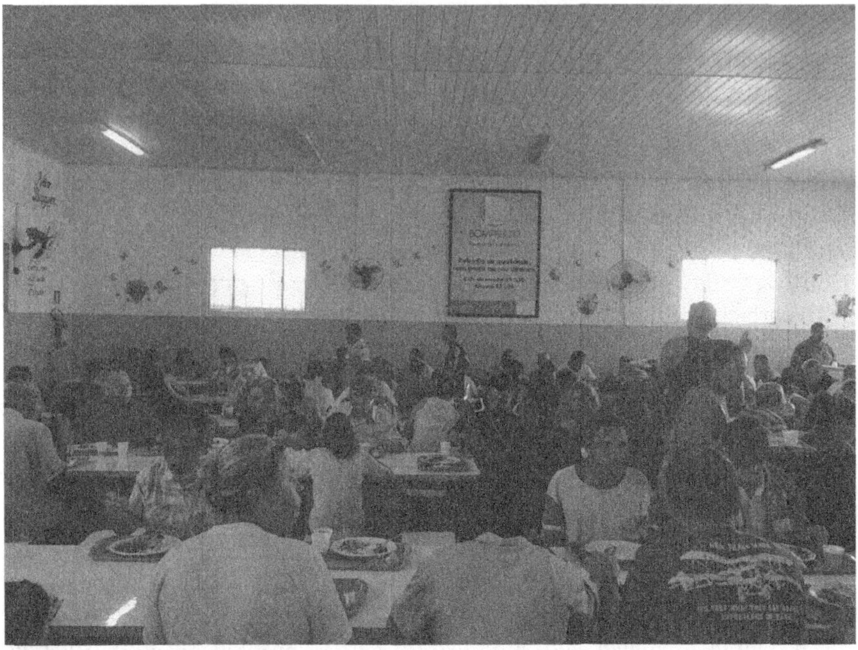

Figure 4.2 Lunch at Bom Prato. *Source*: Photo courtesy of Charles Klein.

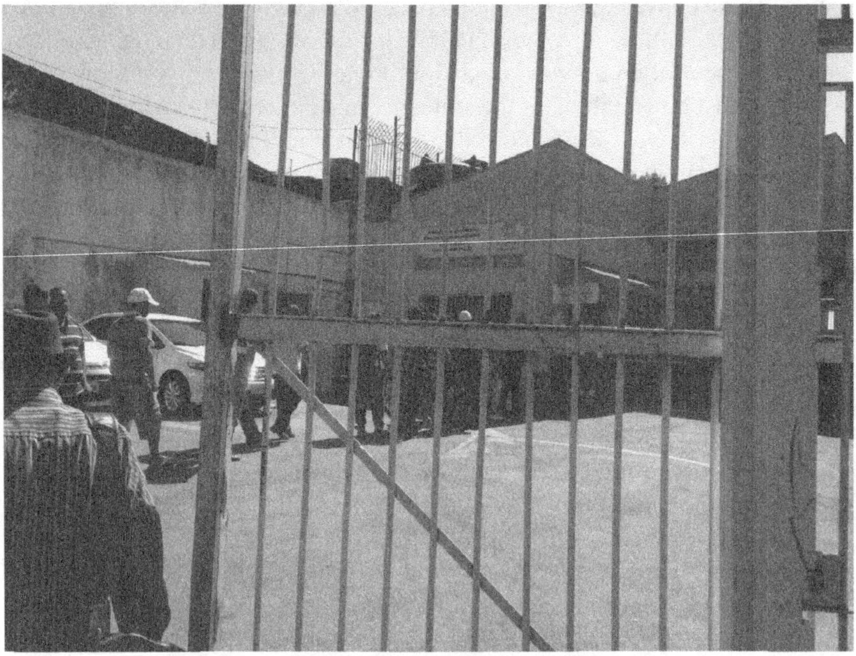

Figure 4.3 Bom Prato lunch line. *Source*: Photo courtesy of Charles Klein.

(Figure 4.3). Around noon, diner demographics shift, with fewer seniors and more working people and families with children. The restaurant stays at capacity and with a line until about 1:15, after which the restaurant gradually empties from 1:30 on. By 2 p.m. closing, Bom Prato has served lunch to 1,400 diners.

Although originally designed to serve economically and socially vulnerable populations, in practice, this restaurant, like most Bom Pratos, serves a cross-section of urban Brazilians. As the case study restaurant manager explains, "some people have a lot of money, some have a moderate income, and some have low or no income" (August 2014 Interview). This cross-class mix, unusual in a sit-down restaurant in Brazil, is a function of the extremely low lunch cost of R$1 (on class segregation in Brazilian cities, see Holston 2008). Most of the lower income customers would not be eating out if the price point were any higher, and for more well-off diners, the savings help them make ends meet in a city with extremely high living costs. Nearly all diners commented favorably on the restaurant's ambience and clientele, and about one-quarter specifically mentioned the cross-class mix as a positive quality, with none saying it is a negative feature.

In terms of food quality, Bom Prato customers gave extremely positive assessments, consistently using adjectives like "good," "marvelous," "high quality," "tasty" and "well prepared." As one diner explained, "Even though the price is low, because the restaurant is directly toward people who are unable to afford eating anywhere else, Bom Prato has the same quality as restaurants with much higher pricing" (26 year-old black male). On the negative side, a few diners suggested that particular dishes might be improved, such as more seasoning in the salad and beans, and several suggested it would be better to serve water or real juice rather than artificially colored "juice-like beverages." A handful also commented that a few staff could serve the food in a more polite manner and that some diners wasted food.

About a third of diners explicitly linked Bom Prato food to healthy or nutritious eating, and a few recounted in detail how Bom Prato had helped them address diet related healthy issues. For example, a 77 year-old white woman explained that "My husband and I had a cholesterol level of over 250, and my husband likes everything fried. At Bom Prato there's nothing like that, and now we have cholesterols below 180. For us it is a blessing to have this here." Another diner highlighted the portions at Bom Prato—"For me, the quantity is right. At other restaurants, they give you a mountain of food that you can't eat without feeling sick. Here, the food is light on the stomach, which for me is good, since I have gastritis" (46 year-old black woman). These narratives affirm the observations of the restaurant manager: "A good thing about eating here is we follow a template, a meal with consistent portions with rice, fruit, juice, salad, etc. And we show that they could follow this model at home too. . . . Customers here tell me that they like to eat here because we follow the guidelines that their doctor set for them" (August 2014 Interview).

LESSONS LEARNED

Over the past three decades, Brazil has developed one of the most fully articulated food and nutritional security paradigms in the world (Kilpatrick 2011). Building on participatory governance forums and substantial state funding, the model has supported innovative initiatives that bridge food production, distribution and eating cultures, including the Bom Prato restaurant network described above. By providing low-cost, freshly prepared meals, Bom Prato makes healthy food daily accessible to tens of thousands of individuals who would otherwise not have the income and/or time to eat a balanced lunch. My case study further suggests that many individuals attempt to follow the general nutritional parameters of the Bom Prato menu in their home cooking and are conscious of the forces that may lead them to less healthy food preparation and eating.

If, as former President Lula argues in the quote at the beginning of this chapter, ending hunger in Brazil requires political will and significant changes in economic policy, the same can be said of reducing rising obesity rates. With its combination of governmental subsidies, healthy meals following national nutritional guidelines, and promotion of traditional food cultures, Bom Prato offers one path for simultaneously supporting obesity prevention and food and nutritional security at the community level. Less clear is whether the Brazilian food and nutritional security movement can expand sufficiently to counter a dominant food system characterized by government supported industrialized agriculture (see, e.g., Brainard 2009; Chaddad and Jank 2006) and the rapid ascension of Big Food (e.g., multinational supermarket chains) and Big Snack (i.e., fast food restaurants) (Monteiro and Cannon 2012). This tension between industrialized food systems and the intersectoral food policy agenda articulated by the National Food and Nutritional Security National Conferences, the CONSEAs, and the 2014 Obesity Prevention and Control Plan can be seen in the sourcing of the food that is served in the Bom Prato restaurant network. Facing the challenges of serving 80,000 healthy meals per day on a budget of R$4-5 (US$1.95–$2.42) per lunch, to date Bom Prato restaurants have sourced product from large-scale, conventional agricultural producers rather than the smaller scale, family farmers in Brazil's cooperative agricultural movement. Bom Prato is, however, initiating two pilot programs in partnership with the *Instituto de Terras de São Paulo* (São Paulo Land Institute/ITESP) that will link family farmers and two Bom Prato restaurants in Sococaba and Rio Claro in the interior of the state of São Paulo. These pilot projects, located in one of Brazil's primary food producing regions, represent important steps in developing alternatives to the large industrialized and processed food sector that has contributed to the rapidly rising obesity rates of the past several decades. Bom Prato program administrators are exploring ways to expand this model to more densely populated areas, such as the capital city of São Paulo. The integration of family farmers within the Bom Prato supply chain would likely require the creation of centralized Bom Prato warehouses (few family farmers in the São Paulo metropolitan region and adjacent areas generate sufficient product to meet the daily needs of a Bom Prato restaurant) and would represent a new direction in program administration (Bom Prato Staff Interview 2014). While local food production initiatives are unlikely to meet the food needs of a megacity like São Paulo, they nonetheless play an important role in affirming that there are real alternatives to industrialized food systems and align with the 2014 São Paulo Master Plan's vision of expanding sustainable, organic agriculture in the city's outer periphery (City of São Paulo 2014). At the consumer level, these programs and policies also demonstrate that it is possible to obtain quality and healthy foods through venues outside of conventional supermarkets and explicitly link healthy eating to community-based, family farms. This growth in alternative food systems is further demonstrated through the nearly 900 street markets registered to operate in the São Paulo (City of São Paulo 2014), including the Feira Do Ibirapuera. This weekly organic market was inaugurated in 2012 at the city's largest and busiest public park and brings together more than 40 organic producers each week. The Feira in turn serves as a central node in an active social media network on Facebook that connects individuals, communities and movements working on food and nutritional security issues throughout Brazil (Feira do Ibiraquera 2015). This growth in both physical farmers markets and online communities suggests that many of the key principles in the food and nutritional paradigm may be coalescing into a cultural movement centered on non-industrialized food system and cultures.

Today, activists and public health practitioners throughout the world are seeking to counter the negative health consequences associated with industrialized food production and the disruption of traditional food cultures. This chapter argues that healthy eating—and by extension obesity prevention—not only requires nutritional directives and behavior change, but also policies and programs such as Brazil's food and nutritional security paradigm that explicitly address the political, economic, and cultural factors that shape eating practices. With our ethnographic toolkit and ability to integrate macro and micro levels of analysis, anthropologists can play a critical role in increasing our understanding of the complex processes through which governmental policies, programs, health-care providers and communities can work together to support healthy food cultures and food systems.

Chapter 5

Metabolic Syndrome Screening and Health Education

Are There Lessons We Can Learn from Japan?

Amy Borovoy

Japan is not the most obvious country from which to gain insight into best practices concerning obesity and public policy. First, Japan has a strikingly low prevalence of obesity: 3.2% of the population, compared with 36.3% in the United States (at the opposite end of the spectrum) and an Organization for Economic Cooperation and Development average of 18.1%. Japan also has a significantly lower prevalence of overweight: 17.9% compared with the OECD average of 28.2% (OECD 2013).[1] While that number is rising, this is occurring more slowly in Japan than in other countries. Perhaps because of lower prevalence, neither the Japanese government nor specific institutions have offered policies specifically related to the problem of obesity.

Yet the Japanese government has been tackling steadily rising population weight through a different platform, one targeting health and lifestyle more broadly rather than simply "weight." The Japanese case is worthy of study as an example of approaching population weight as an encompassing issue of cultural values, beliefs, health, and lifestyle. In some sense this resonates with health-centered approaches that are gaining attention in the United States which decenter weight loss in favor of an emphasis on sustainable norms, general health, and moderate physical activity.[2] It is also resonant with recent behavioral models of health that encourage individuals to make better choices by strategically modifying the environment—in the interest of avoiding more regulatory (and hence paternalistic) measures such as taxation, marketing, or use restrictions. Yet the question the Japan comparison raises is whether these more measured, "lifestyle" approaches can be effective in the absence of the powerful role that Japanese family, schools, health care, and workplaces play in promoting social norms that guide daily life. In this sense the "health-oriented" approach to obesity may be less transferrable to other places—particularly the U. S., where public health and preventative health mandates are a thinner presence in daily life.

Japan is distinguished by its positive public health environment: socio-economic factors that influence population health, including relative income inequality, low levels of violent crime, a relatively healthy food environment despite pervasive Westernization of diet, and modes of commuting that rely on walking and biking to public transportation. In addition, medical services for individuals in the form of preventative care, education, and screening are widely accessible and affordable, and because Japanese citizens visit doctors relatively frequently, health messages and education are integrated into everyday life. Thus, the Japanese system provides not only "health care" but also what we might call "health consciousness" (R. Campbell 1996; Lock 1997, 208; Reich et al. 2011; Reid 2009, 84).

In what follows I highlight the role of mass screening, education, and preventative care in Japanese medicine, as exemplified by Japan's recent initiative to screen all citizens between the ages of 40 and 74 for metabolic syndrome. The policy mandates the weighing and measurement of adults between these ages and emphasizes counseling and education as a way to encourage citizens to make healthier choices.

In considering what we might learn from the Japan's policies and what role anthropologists might play in formulating policy in response to obesity, I draw on earlier research concerning the implementation of the screening policy in corporate settings, and how Japan's approach to curbing population weight gain and chronic illness might help us think beyond the juxtaposition that U.S. policy-makers often invoke between "individual responsibility" and "environmental regulation" (Borovoy and Roberto 2015). I also draw on my recent research concerning Japan's public health measures more broadly and the emphasis placed on health education in spheres beyond health care.

The screening policy was initially implemented in 2008 as part of a broader set of initiatives mandated in Japan's Health Promotion Law *(Kenkō Zōshin H),* passed in 2002 and implemented beginning in 2003. One measure of the law was to extend the purpose of citizens' yearly physical exam from diagnosing disease to addressing issues of lifestyle more broadly. Japan's screening program may not offer an example of best practices that can be easily embraced in other societies. However, it raises important questions about the role that social norms and everyday institutions play in maintaining population health. It also raises the question of the policy implications of targeting "pre-clinical conditions" or "syndromes" as objects of intervention. These are groups of physiological conditions that indicate heightened future risk of chronic illness. Diagnosing such syndromes heightens awareness and may encourage behavioral change, but it also medicalizes bodily conditions that may be presently asymptomatic, potentially paving the way for preliminary medical or pharmaceutical interventions.

In considering the implications of screening for metabolic syndrome as a means of promoting health, it is important to note that metabolic syndrome is not a "disease"; individuals are usually asymptomatic and do not experience impediments to leading a normal life. It is, rather, a cluster of conditions, including elevated blood sugar, blood pressure, and cholesterol, and excess fat around the waist associated with insulin resistance. For those with metabolic syndrome, cells in the body do not respond to insulin, the hormone produced by the pancreas that allows cells to absorb glucose; thus glucose levels rise in the body. Metabolic syndrome is a concern because it is associated with later risk of chronic illness, such as diabetes, cardiovascular disease, and stroke. Though metabolic syndrome can be caused by obesity, it is often described as the "pre-clinical stage" or "borderline" state before metabolic issues result in diabetes, hypertension, obesity, or cardiovascular disease. Thus, insulin resistance is associated with being overweight and with lifestyle factors such as inactivity, but it is not equivalent to obesity or overweight. The "special examination" *(tokutei kenkō shinsa)* imposed by the new law requires blood sugar, pressure, and cholesterol tests, in addition to a measurement of the circumference around the belly button. While "thickened waist" is regarded as one index of metabolic syndrome; obesity itself is not the focus of this policy. Treatment for metabolic syndrome focuses on lifestyle change more broadly, with diet as one aspect.[3]

The Japanese Ministry of Health, Labor, and Welfare's encompassing Health Promotion Law is a long-term program aimed at cutting costs that the government will likely face in the coming decades due to its rapidly aging population. The Ministry hopes that metabolic syndrome screening will, over the long term, reduce the incidence of costly chronic illness among the aging population, and thereby relieve the state's growing financial burden of health care for the elderly. In contrast with policies designed to address the already advanced problem of obesity in the United States, for example, this is a preventative strategy, aimed largely at curbing future costs.

THE METABOLIC SYNDROME SCREENING PROGRAM

It is important to note that the Ministry has taken a "soft" approach to containing rising population weight. Interventions prescribed for those diagnosed with metabolic syndrome or pre-metabolic "warning signs" focus on counseling, education, and support. What the Japanese Ministry of Health is *not* proposing is the imposition of stronger regulatory measures on harm-producing industries (food, tobacco, or liquor). Public health activists and policy-minded scholars in the United States have increasingly emphasized the need to reform the food environment, as research has illuminated the role of food marketing, portion sizes, and other external factors in influencing individual choices (Borovoy and Roberto 2015; Institute of Medicine 2012).

In contrast, the metabolic screening and counseling program offers an easily accessible, well-supervised support and education program. Metabolic syndrome screening and counseling calls on individuals to make better choices through moderation, endurance, patience, self-control, record-keeping, and the reliance on family members for support. The pamphlets and guidelines (detailed below) emphasize incremental improvement and good common sense, providing basic nutritional and lifestyle advice. While the advice is prudent, the burden for health maintenance is placed squarely on the shoulders of the individual. Smoking cessation, sufficient exercise and sleep, eating in moderation—all are seen as habits that the individual can control with the right strategies and appropriate knowledge.

The Mayo Clinic describes "aggressive lifestyle changes" as the appropriate treatment for metabolic syndrome, including exercise, healthful eating, and smoking cessation. The Ministry of Health has embraced the agenda of lifestyle reform, targeting its PR campaign to address a broad range of issues, including family life, urban planning, sports promotion, in the endeavor to produce a society in which "every citizen can achieve a fulfilling lifestyle" (*kokumin ga kokoro yūtaka ni seikatsu dekiru)* (Japan Ministry of Health 2009, 65–66). Educational pamphlets produced by the Ministry, local government health center, and insurance organizations describe metabolic syndrome, diabetes, liver disease, and cardiovascular disease as "diseases of the lifestyle" *(seikatsu shūkanbyō)*. In treatment interventions and educational materials, emphasis is placed on diet, exercise, rest, and curbing consumption of alcohol and tobacco. "Lifestyle improvement" (*seikatsu shūkan kaizen),* "guidance" *(shidō),* "support" *(shien),* "prevention" *(yobō),* and "health management" *(kenkō kanri)* are key terms associated with the metabolic syndrome screening program.

Pamphlets produced by the Ministry, health insurance organizations, and community health centers *(hokenjo)* are dense with specific information, yet they are highly accessible and user-friendly, with cartoon-style graphics and illustrations, space for self-reporting, and smiling, upbeat images of counselors and advisors. The pamphlets offer highly specific nutritional guidelines (e.g., "Eat at least 350 grams of vegetables each day: 120 grams green vegetable and 330 colored"), BMI calculators, calorie calculators, breakfast lunch and dinner menus with recipes including calorie and nutrient lists, exercise regimens and calorie counters, diagrams of appropriate posture and ergonomics for sitting and exercise, illustrations of appropriate daily intake, and so forth (e.g., Kanagawa Prefecture 2010; Meiji Yasuda 2009). Advice promoted in these educational pamphlets includes:

- Wait three minutes when you feel the urge to eat in between meals [to see if it passes].
- Do your daily chores vigorously *(sekkyokuteki)*.
- Get off the train or bus early in order to walk a 15-minute portion of your daily commute.
- Take the stairs rather than elevator or escalator for up to three floors to get to your office.
- Chew food about 30 times (by your estimate) before swallowing.
- Drink alcohol in "appropriate" amounts *(tekiryō)* [appropriate amounts of various alcoholic beverages are specified].
- Limit canned coffee to one a day [canned coffee is a popular, sugary drink in Japan sold ubiquitously in vending machines].

The Ministry has yet to release aggregated data on whether the interventions are working (the first 5-year trial run was completed in 2015), and any data are preliminary as the Ministry's chief concern is long-term savings through preventative care. While we cannot yet estimate the effectiveness of the screening program alone, it is important to note that the screening operates within a broader social context in which health concerns and health education are integrated into non-health institutions, such as school, and companies. Furthermore, health is closely linked to other social values concerning comportment, hygiene, regularity of life habits, sharing and sociality, manners, and specific beliefs about food, such as the privileging of Japanese food and of small quantities as particularly tasty and high in quality. While the program focuses solely on life habits rather than environmental interventions and heavily places the burden of lifestyle reform on the individual, it relies on existing institutions to support behavioral change and to perpetuate social norms that are conducive to health.

Some have argued that the focus on life habits is a welcome departure from the medicalization of obesity as an illness in itself, a trend that has supported the treatment of obesity through medical interventions and fad diets, and reified the problem as its own distinct ailment (and "cause" of other chronic illnesses) rather than as a symptom of shared patterns of unhealthy behavioral patterns (Oliver 2006, 8–11).

Factors Affecting Implementation of and Compliance with Metabolic Syndrome Screening

Company insurance organizations exert a powerful influence over employees because of the employee's close relationship to the company, forged through a range of welfare provisions including family expenses, housing, recreation, sick leave, and pensions. Health insurance coverage for citizens was put in place in the early twentieth century with the agenda of nation-building in mind. The program expanded rapidly before and during World War II in the endeavor to produce "healthy people and healthy soldiers" and retained strong support after the war, resulting in complete coverage in 1961 (Ikegami and Maeda 2014; Campbell, Ikegami, and Tsugawa 2104, 18–19). Japan's system of universal coverage has made health care comprehensive, accessible, and affordable, meaning that health care is a pervasive and powerful in shaping daily life.

Employers are the largest overseers of health insurance in Japan. Insurance is provided by health insurance organizations *(kenkō hoken kumiai),* which are closely affiliated with the company, covered through a payroll tax. Employers also contribute to costs in varying amounts. Large companies, who receive no government subsidy for health care provision, often have clinics on-site, and firms with over 700 employees have their own public health nurses, who are trained by the government as civil servants. Some firms even maintain large hospitals for their employees (Reid 2009, 86). Companies employ public health nurses to implement the screening program, and because the public health nurse is known throughout the company and the program is closely affiliated with the workplace (sometimes even on the premises), employee health organizations are potentially an effective means of communicating health messages and eliciting compliance with the Ministry's prescribed behavior (Borovoy and Roberto 2015).

According to Ministry of Health mandates, those who show warning signs of metabolic syndrome must undergo two sessions of counseling and education called "motivational support" (*dōkizuke shien*). The counseling sessions take place either at a contracted institution or, in larger companies with an on-site clinic, at the place of one's employment with a public health nurse. Those diagnosed with metabolic syndrome must undergo "enthusiastic support" (*sekkyoku teki shien)* for six months with a six-month follow up for "self-reflection" *(furikae).*

Ministry of Health guidelines for these interventions are precise. "Motivational support" sessions include 80 minutes of group counseling, 20 minutes of individual counseling, and a six-month follow-up. "Enthusiastic support" includes the same rounds of counseling, two mail or phone follow-ups two weeks and one month later respectively, one five-minute phone call two months after, plus one 20-minute interview three months later, and finally, one five-minute phone call six months later to follow-up. While the screening itself is folded into the yearly battery of recommended exams, the follow-up counseling has required new infrastructure. The insurance organization associated with Shimomura Electronics, one company I visited, reported spending approximately 2.5 million dollars per year on the counseling interventions alone (Borovoy and Roberto 2015).

The Ministry of Health, Labor, and Welfare has placed a heavy burden on health insurance organizations, which bear the cost of implementing the metabolic syndrome screening program for the majority of the population. In addition, the Ministry has threatened to fine companies who do not show improvement in rates of metabolic syndrome or pre-metabolic syndrome—though I have not been able to find out exactly how much improvement is required. (Nor have I identified any instances in which this fine as actually levied; it seems to be more a "guideline" or a threat than a policy.) Nonetheless, public health concerns as well as other related issues (such as mental health issues—a growing area of awareness) are increasingly seen as included in the large-scale enterprise's welfare package *(fukurikōsei)*. There is a conflict of interest here that deserves further study. Since the corporate culture of long hours and after-hours drinking (understood to contribute to camaraderie in business relations) likely contributes to rising rates of metabolic syndrome and chronic illness, how effective will the Ministry of Health's message program be? How do employees respond to these conflicting demands and balance the desire for good health with the demands of the workplace? How do managers respond when their subordinates leave early to get adequate rest, or decline to join in for after-hours drinking?

ACCESSIBILITY OF HEALTH CARE

In addition to the links between workplace and health care, Japan's health care system itself has created a culture in which citizens frequently visit the doctor. Citizens are required to be insured through one within a range of non-profit insurance plans, some of which are independent (insurance organizations affiliated with large firms) and others which are subsidized by the national government (those for employees of smaller companies, the self-employed, retirees and others). Tight government regulation and the imposition of a single, universal fee schedule for procedures, surgeries, and doctors' visits, make health care affordable. As a result, Japanese citizens visit doctors more frequently (approximately 14.5 times a year on average, though this number is skewed by the rapidly growing number of elderly; the average number for Japanese citizens over age 65 is about 26 times a year) (Campbell and Ikegami 1998; Reid 2009, 84; R. Campbell 1996, 227). Thus, the Japanese system fosters health awareness through frequent visits for routine ailments, combined with an aggressive and comprehensive public mass screening program.

Tests included in this program, while varying year-to-year according to Ministry of Health recommendations, are: health history, height, weight, waist measurement, blood pressure, blood tests for liver function, cholesterol, and creatinine, urinalysis, heart and lung exam, and additional tests if indicated by initial results. While the basic exam is not particularly extensive, the pressure upon citizens to comply with yearly check-ups is more intense than in the United States, where insurance is usually private (with the exception of Medicare, Medicaid, and veterans' medicine) and for-profit. In addition, some companies and insurance plans subsidize more comprehensive yearly exams. These exams, known as "human dry docks" *(ningen dokku),* include extensive and invasive testing and measurement, including stomach and intestinal X-rays (barium enema and sometimes endoscopy), hearing tests, chest X-ray, family health history and lifestyle questionnaire, complete blood count, and certain cancer screenings. While screening is costly and potentially wasteful, some have argued that this vigilance about health and awareness of the body has contributed to Japan's positive health outcomes in part because it makes Japanese patients more well-educated and aware of health symptoms and risks (Campbell and Ikegami 1998; Yukawa et al. 2010).

"Health education" is also integrated into other spheres of daily life in Japan. Japan has a comprehensive school lunch program that covers almost all elementary schools and many middle schools. The school lunch program was founded in 1872 in conjunction with making elementary school compulsory for all citizens. From the start, school lunches were conceptualized as pedagogical devices that could educate students about proper nutrition, as well as manners, comportment, hygiene, and the importance of limiting waste. School lunches are mandatory (children are not allowed to bring food from home), and lunchtime is regarded as an educational moment: children eat in classrooms, ingredients of school lunches are regulated by the Ministry of Education, and eating lunch is regarded as an opportunity to socialize children about appropriate calorie intake, balanced meals, and nutrition—in addition to manners, hygiene, limiting waste, and sometimes education about local foods, aesthetics, and ceramic ware (Borovoy and Roberto 2015; McLemore 2015; Suginami Ward 2012). Schools have historically assumed responsibility for weighing children each month, as well as for supervising dental care. Thus, health and the body are regarded as aspects of education in Japan (Ohnuki-Tierney 1984).

It is also important to note that by many measures, Japanese citizens form one of the healthiest populations in the world. Although the divide between the wealthy and poor has grown and the level of poverty has risen in the past 20 years, infant mortality is still relatively low; life expectancy is high; few children are born to single parents; and even after two decades of dramatically slowed economic growth, unemployment is low. Crime rates are still relatively low, the Japanese diet is healthful (although less healthful foreign foods have made significant inroads into daily consumption), and urban Japanese citizens are less sedentary due to their reliance on public transportation.

Thus, the metabolic syndrome screening program, which emphasizes bodily awareness, self-control, and healthy living habits, takes place in a context in which citizens are already relatively healthy, and secondary institutions can support messages offered by the Ministry of Health through the screening program and yearly check-ups (Lock 1997, 208; Reich et al. 2011).

WEIGHING THE TRADE-OFFS OF METABOLIC SYNDROME SCREENING: WHAT, IF ANYTHING, CAN WE LEARN FROM JAPAN?

In the United States, public health activists have had to fight against the assumption that health and weight loss rest on individual, freely-made choices. The assumption has been that responsibility for becoming obese resides with poor choices made by the individual (Kersh 2009). But the model of "individual free choice" is highly problematic in a context in which consumers are heavily manipulated by a food industry that many would argue is under-regulated. In the past decade, public health researchers have illuminated the role of environmental factors that drive obesity, including food marketing, the availability of inexpensive, nutrient-poor, and calorie-dense foods, large portion sizes, as well as declining physical activity, social networks and neighborhood environments (Christakis and Fowler 2007; Eisenberg this volume). Some scholars have suggested that environmental factors associated with obesity are so overwhelming that it is unrealistic to expect individuals to consistently make healthy decisions (Benson 2014; Bonell et al. 2011; Brownell et al. 2010). While public health initiatives such as Michelle Obama's "Let's Move" campaign continue to attempt to raise awareness among consumers concerning appropriate diet and exercise, many public health researchers have increasingly advocated policy changes that target environmental drivers of obesity such as taxing sugary drinks, banning vending machines in schools, and restricting child-targeted advertising—moves which seek to limit consumer choice (Kersh and Morone 2002, 151).

The Japanese government has not followed this lead. The government continues to be strong on education and consciousness-raising and relatively weak on imposing restrictions on harmful products such as tobacco, and in regulating harm industries through taxation, limits on advertising, or mandated labels. For example, Japan Tobacco is a government-run monopoly. The smoking ordinance passed under Health Promotion Law implemented in 2003 is still ambiguous, requiring hospitals, schools, gyms, theaters, department stores, and other public spaces to take "necessary measures" *(hitsuyō na sochi)* to prevent the inhalation of passive smoke. In 2002 Chiyoda Ward became the first ward to ban smoking on busy streets, and other wards have created smoking areas. Many public spaces and institutions impose smoking bans as private measures, and social pressure and slowly growing awareness of the damage of passive smoke have pushed people to comply with smoking segregation in the absence of firmer regulations (Feldman 2001). In sum, as Christina Roberto and I have argued, key aspects of Japan's "softer" approach to paternalism consist of (1) the pervasive and persuasive linkage between health and daily life habits; (2) an emphasis on self-regulation with support; and (3) the implementation of social norms through institutions such as health care, schools, and companies, and families (2015).

Recently, alternatives to state-based paternalism have received attention in the United States as attempts to guard against the potential failure of educational efforts. These are described by behavioral economists as "libertarian paternalism," or "nudging." In their best-selling book, *Nudge: Improving Decisions About Health, Wealth, and Happiness* (2008), economist Richard Thaler and University of Chicago legal theorist Cass Sunstein (a former appointee in the Obama administration Office of Information and Regulatory Affairs) advocate preserving individual freedom through "nudging" individuals to make better choices by making these choices easier. For example, "nudging" means not banning vending machines or sweet desserts from school cafeterias, but rather "putting the fruit at eye level" (Thaler and Sunstein 2008, 6). Thaler and Sunstein claim that they are helping individuals to make the choices that they themselves would prefer to make—making healthy decisions easier. Their environmental interventions help individuals who suffer from cognitive biases such as "optimism," short-term planning, or temptation to reach positive outcomes anyway, by making "default" alternatives more helpful (for example, requiring individuals to "opt out" of 401(k) accounts rather than "opt in").

Thaler and Sunstein hope to capture the best of both worlds—allowing freedom of choice while encouraging healthful behavior. It is noteworthy that Thaler and Sunstein make no claims to shaping the way people think. They eschew that idea, preferring instead to modify the environment without having to alter core beliefs and values (2008). (This is in contrast with Japan's intense emphasis on socio-cultural beliefs and socialization.) "Nudging" depends on specific interventions which purport to be agnostic or at least non-coercive in encouraging individuals to make specific choices. However, one wonders how effective such piecemeal interventions can be in a climate like the U.S. where there is less consensus around social norms, it is more difficult to set nationally shared standards for healthy body metrics, and institutions such as health care and education are less closely dictated by state mandates. Consequently, the legal regulation of advertising, presentation, and use of commercial products, neighborhood zoning, and taxation may have a stronger role to play (Borovoy and Roberto 2015; Eisenberg this volume).

Indeed, public health activists in Japan have pushed for legal restrictions of harm industries such as the tobacco industry. Where the state has failed to implement stronger regulations, owing in part to close relationships with large-scale industrial interests, the deployment of social norms has been a secondary measure (Feldman 2001). With respect to metabolic syndrome, the Ministry of Health is in some ways promoting conflicting messages, for example by failing to regulate tobacco advertising while supporting tobacco cessation education in the context of corporate health care. One might say something similar with respect to attitudes towards over-work, a precipitant of some of Japan's key public health issues, including metabolic syndrome.

METABOLIC SYNDROME AS CATEGORY

Nonetheless, the attention to lifestyle promoted by metabolic syndrome is worth considering in efforts at public health promotion outside of Japan. Interventions targeting metabolic syndrome are more preventative, more inclusive, and more wide-ranging in their recommendations than policies aimed strictly at obesity. With a totalizing emphasis on "health" rather than a targeted emphasis on "obesity," citizens do not have to identify as obese, overweight, or even as unhealthy in order to subscribe to the policy recommendations. Metabolic syndrome is seen in Japan as a phenomenon that could affect anyone, and is explicitly linked with middle-class lifestyles, including long commute times, Westernization of food, overwork, excessive consumption of alcohol and tobacco, and poor sleep hygiene.

It is possible that the category of metabolic syndrome screening could help avoid the medicalization of obesity by focusing on lifestyle and prevention, rather than treating obesity after the fact through a heavy reliance on medical solutions, including bariatric surgery or weight loss drugs that may diminish the behavioral and lifestyle issues that precipitated the problem (Oliver 2006, 8–10). Some have argued that medical procedures are over-prescribed in a culture of medical entrepreneurship, while basic health care in the form of prevention, lifestyle, sidewalks, and diet management is overlooked. As a result the Japanese Ministry of Health has recognized the value of focusing on lifestyle.

However, there are concerns associated with diagnosing "pre-clinical" conditions or "syndromes" (Mitka 2005). In an essay on "the turn to chronic disease" in global health, Ian Whitmarsh cautions, "With chronic diseases, the locus of intervention shifts from attempting to remove structural barriers or expand access to medications to convincing individuals to see themselves as ill or potentially ill and to act accordingly . . ." (2013, 303).

Interventions target individual behavior; and they target individuals before they are symptomatic. Indeed the government has not only identified "metabolic syndrome" as an object of treatment; it has also defined "pre-metabolic syndrome" as a status that requires intervention.[4] Here the trade-offs need to be weighed carefully. While preventative care can be valuable, treating preconditions opens doors to the pharmaceutical industry to target "symptoms" and "precursors" rather than "illnesses."

Indeed, the American Diabetes Association has already expressed concerns about the use of the diagnosis, worrying that the diagnosis implies that the "syndrome" carries a greater risk than individual risk factors, and that it is a distraction from recommendations for "prediabetic" patients, for whom recommended interventions are more stringent than those for metabolic syndrome. However, proponents of the category, including the U.S. National Heart, Lung, and Blood Institute (NHLBI), argue that the diagnosis is useful in directing individual patients to address their risk factors. They assert that the label directs attention to the necessary issue of lifestyle change and moves treatment away from the "drug approach" that informs the treatment of individual risk factors (Mitka 2005, 13).

Recognizing metabolic syndrome as a treatment category could expand the target population of those who need care. Metabolic syndrome recognizes a broader spectrum of health issues and promotes a wider range of interventions, including non-medical interventions. The broader conceptualization of "health" offered in the metabolic syndrome approach decenters the issue of "weight" and privileges the importance of life habits, including self-care, relaxation, cooking, eating at home, basic nutrition, sleep, and basic health care. It is compatible with the move to "de-medicalize health," a move that has been called for by policy analysts (Brownlee 2008; Gawande 2009). Demedicalizing health and placing obese and non-obese persons in one single category subject to a unified program of intervention could also potentially diminish the stigma associated with obesity.

Culture and social institutions shape the range of options available for any society to confront the problem of rising rates of chronic illness, overweight, and obesity. The Japan example reveals to us how far the effects of social institutions such as schools and primary level health care can stretch, even in the context of relatively weak industry regulations. It is unlikely that the imposition of a single, standardized regime of appropriate lifestyle habits and body metrics would be embraceable in societies that do not possess the supportive institutions of Japanese corporate welfare, universal health care, and nation-wide school pedagogy around health and nutrition. Still, Japan's socio-cultural approach suggests that anthropologists will have a powerful role to play in the analysis necessary to reach better solutions globally.

NOTES

1. According to WHO classifications, obesity is defined as BMI greater than 30. Overweight is defined as a BMI between 25 and 30. (The data is taken from 2010 or latest available.)

2. For example, the growing "Health at Every Size" paradigm, which de-emphasizes weight loss as the single barometer of health and instead emphasizes "intuitive eating," body acceptance, and exercise for health rather than elite performance or body shape (Penney and Kirk 2015).

3. In Japan metabolic syndrome is defined as:

Waist (belly) measurement ≥ 85 cm (men) ≥ 90 cm for women (In the United States the measurements are slightly different: ≥ 102 cm (men) and ≥ 89 cm (women))

AND two (or more) of the below three conditions:

1. Triglycerides (TG) ≥ 150mg/dl **and/or** HDL cholesterol < 40 mg/dl
2. Systolic blood pressure ≥ 130mmHg **and/or** diastolic blood pressure ≥ 85mmHg
3. Blood sugar (fasting) ≥ 110mg/dl (U.S. 100 mg/dl)

4. Pre-metabolic syndrome or "warning signs" are defined as waist size larger than prescribed plus any one of the three conditions of elevated triglycerides, blood pressure, or blood sugar (see endnote 3).

Chapter 6

Who, What, and How?[1]

Insights Gained From a Comparative Approach to School-Based Obesity Prevention Efforts

Alexandra G. Lancey

Childhood obesity is one of the most significant health problems facing the United States today. Since 1980, the prevalence of obesity in children aged 6–19 years has tripled, and these children often face heightened risk of diseases such as Type II diabetes and cardiovascular disease, diminished quality of life, and premature death (Li and Hooker 2010). In 2012, the Centers for Disease Control and Prevention reported that 17% of youth and 34.9% of adults were obese. Though the prevalence of obesity has remained relatively stable in recent years, a persistent belief is that the incidence of obesity among Americans will continue to rise (Ogden et al. 2014). In Virginia, where one part of our case study takes place, the most recent statistics from the CDC indicate that 27.2% of adults are obese. Furthermore, in 2011 14.3% of Virginia's children (aged 10–17) were obese, and almost 30% were overweight or obese (State of Obesity 2012).

Worldwide, obesity and overweight are becoming some of the most threatening health concerns of our time, especially among children. Since 1980, the World Health Organization (WHO) (2013) reports, global childhood obesity rates have also tripled in many countries, with 170 million children (aged 17 and under) overweight in 2012. This growth is concerning globally, but certain countries are experiencing the epidemic more severely than others. The Western Pacific region is especially affected, with adult obesity rates of over 60% in many countries (Gani 2009). In particular, the Republic of Palau (the other half of our case study), a Pacific island nation of about 20,000 people, declared a state of emergency due to the growing obesity epidemic in 2011 (Kuartei 2011). The obesity rate was almost 60% for adults, and 33% for school aged children in 2011, and these numbers are on the rise (Kuartei 2011). Mounting obesity in the Republic of Palau has been linked by various studies to increasing pressures from modernization and the effects of globalization (Cassels 2006; Duerler and Maskarinec 2007; Engleberger et al. 2005; Jabre 1981; Kermode and Tellei 2005; Labarthe et al. 1973; Pobocik et al. 2000). Engleberger et al. (2005) discuss the trend in Pacific culture to disregard local foods and local food production as "low status," while the imported foods provided to countries like Palau (mainly from Japan and the United States) are more desirable and impressive in a social context. Additionally, imported "convenience foods" have made up the majority of the Palauan diet for much of the last half of the twentieth century, and today seem to fit better with changing times, characterized by urbanization and a more faced-paced lifestyle (Kermode and Tellei 2005). Yet, these convenience foods are often higher in fat and calories and lower in nutritional value (Cassels 2006).

Palau has been significantly influenced by the United States since World War II, but has a distinct cultural background and far different place in the global economic scheme. Still, many of their growing concerns surrounding obesity and lifestyle-related non-communicable diseases, a trend toward overconsumption of calorie-dense convenience foods and a more sedentary lifestyle are not unlike those we see in the United States Additionally, the political and historical factors influencing school nutrition decision making in Palau (as a result of feeling economically beholden to larger world powers) are not unlike to differences in wealth and power in various communities throughout the U.S. that leave them unable or unwelcome in expressing their opinions, needs, and challenges when federally-funded programs are handed down (Crooks 2003).

Comparing two different approaches in public schools in these countries allows anthropologists to better understand which aspects of nutrition education approaches and efforts to promote healthy eating are limited by culture, and which can be generalized to contribute to greater theoretical explanations, which can then be conveyed to policymakers, school officials, and other stakeholders involved in school nutrition education programming across the world. Further, because of the differences in approach between the two countries in light of their similarities, there are successful elements of school nutrition education and ways of overcoming barriers that can ultimately be shared and developed on a national or international scale. This chapter describes a case study in two mid-size, urban, public elementary schools: one in the Palau, and one in a Southwest Virginia community aimed at exploring what community-driven efforts were in place at each school to combat childhood obesity and educate children about healthy eating.

OBESITY PREVENTION AND INTERVENTION IN SCHOOLS

As childhood obesity has become a central focus in Palauan and American public health efforts, schools have surfaced as important venues for investigating the disease and for attempts at intervention and prevention. Importantly, studies link childhood overweight and obesity with poor academic performance, citing lower standardized test scores, behavioral problems, and low attendance rates as key concerns that can be improved with better nutrition (Burkhalter and Hillman 2011; Hollar et al. 2010). Moreover, these cognitive performance concerns often continue into adulthood, leading to decreased mental and intellectual performance and ability in the workplace (Burkhalter and Hillman 2011). School nutrition has been a key focus of policymakers due in part to the fact that children consume a large portion of their daily food intake at school. School serves as the primary venue for learning about nutrition and modeling positive nutrition-related behaviors. In other words, schools assist mightily in conveying localized foodways and norms to students. Therefore, not surprisingly, many scholars have concluded that schools are ideal places for implementing policies and programs that seek to improve nutrition and combat obesity, but further research is necessary to determine best practices for such activities to determine what is deemed to be most effective at improving nutrition in schools, changing nutritional behavior at home, and improving academic performance.

In recent years, public health and nutrition scholars have looked to schools as a key location for nutrition education. Most of this work is evaluative in nature. Public health and nutrition experts often focus on evaluating specific programs or policies put in place by nonprofits, coalitions, or local and state government agencies. These studies have involved specific programs and specific (mostly quantitative) measured outcomes. For example, Probart and colleagues studied a Pennsylvania program designed to help school food service personnel and administrators strategize and work to improve school environments and school food, while providing small grants to help with assessment and development (2007). The authors of this study assisted in this evaluation using, interestingly enough, qualitative in-depth interview methods. Major barriers to improving school food environments in the 22 schools interviewed in this Pennsylvania study included time and money, communication, adult skepticism, and student involvement/ownership.

Other studies have looked more specifically into programs designed for smaller or special populations. Craven's (2011) study looked specifically at ninth graders in rural high schools that were enrolled in a health class. The class "received 6 hours of nutrition education based on social cognitive theory" (2011, 141). They measured the success of the program in overall BMI change and reported fruit and vegetable intake, and concluded that a required health class, then, could be an effective method for change. Hollar and colleagues (2009) conducted a similar study that studied the effects of a specific intervention that both attempted to bring nutrition foods and incorporate healthy eating information curricula to low income elementary students. The authors of this study, too, used BMI measures to determine whether this kind of intervention could be successful with their specific population. These studies have helped researchers and school officials, in collaboration with community partners, develop more effective programming for different student populations. Additionally, this work has fortified the understanding that there may not be a one-size-fits-all approach to this kind of prevention and intervention programming. Building on this work, we wanted to develop an approach that used qualitative methods to understand what parents and teachers felt made programs or policies successful and better understand not just the outcomes of certain school programs on student BMI overtime, but get a better idea of the experiences parents and teachers had with their students while implementing these programs and policies. What makes school-based obesity prevention efforts successful? What can parent and teacher experiences tell us about the efficacy and sustainability of these efforts? How can a cross-cultural comparative study help us answer these questions more effectively?

A COMPARATIVE CASE STUDY: PUBLIC ELEMENTARY SCHOOLS IN TWO CITIES

Our research was designed to examine the questions above by querying parents of children at each school to understand attitudes toward the programs and learn about how these programs were influencing nutritional behavior change in their children. We also wanted to use a comparative approach (Sobal 1998) that built on applied anthropological research and program design methods to help us pinpoint key assets and barriers to nutrition education and to speak to greater implications for such programs at other schools in hopes of seeking means of more effectively combining these two approaches in future research.

Data Collection in Koror

The Palau portion of this research focuses on Koror Elementary School, a K-8 school in Ngerbeched, an urban neighborhood located in Palau's population center ("KES" henceforth). Two mixed-method surveys were constructed for parents and teachers. The surveys combined both quantitative and qualitative questions about school food, child nutritional habits, academic performance, and opinions regarding school nutrition policies and programs. All teachers at the school received the survey from the principal. Parents were given the survey at a Parent Teacher Association meeting, which, of note, usually has parental attendance rates exceeding 50%. Data analysis took place using SPSS software for the quantitative survey questions, and coding/thematic analysis for the qualitative questions. A total of 167 respondents completed the survey (33 teachers and 134 parents). Twenty-seven female and 6 male teachers were surveyed, and 90 female and 41 male parents (3 respondents did not indicate gender).

In addition, three interviews were conducted, by phone, with Palauan teachers and school officials. These interviews were used to provide contextual detail to augment interpretation of survey data.

Southwest Virginia Data Collection

The U.S. portion of the study focuses on a mid-size urban K-5 school in Roanoke, Virginia ("VES" henceforth). Survey formation and distribution was completed as part of an ongoing study. Parents were given a mixed-method survey that combined both quantitative and qualitative questions about school food, child nutritional habits, academic performance, and opinions regarding the school's current policies and programs. Surveys were sent home with students (grades K-5) as a homework assignment from their physical education teacher. Students were asked to complete the surveys with their parents at home and return them to the teacher. Data analysis took place as above. A total of 83 parents completed the survey with their children.

PARENT AND TEACHER PERCEPTIONS OF SCHOOL-BASED NUTRITION EDUCATION

The data shared below are insights and ideas from parents and teachers at both study sites. These data can be construed as evidence of the strengths and weaknesses of two different approaches to school nutrition education programming and policymaking. Both study sites have different programs in place (in the case of KES: policies that prevent students from bringing unhealthy snacks or sweetened beverages, as well as some school gardening programs; at VES, some coalition-run programs that mostly consist of cooking demonstrations and discussions of healthy eating learning how to prepare healthy foods).

Targeting Specific Behaviors

One of the survey questions asked about nutritional behavior of students at home with their parents. First, the survey asked how often parents participated in various healthy eating activities with their children. Possible responses included assisting with cooking at home, grocery shopping, trying new foods, and reading nutrition labels. At both KES and VES, parents most often reported grocery shopping together with their children, and the least common activity was reading nutrition labels.

Then, parents were given a list of activities related to nutrition (such as reading nutrition labels, discussing healthy eating with friends, and choosing healthier snacks), and were asked to define whether or not they had seen this change in their child as a result of the programs or policies in place at each study site. In both Palau and Southwest Virginia, one of the most frequent changes in behavior was choosing healthier snacks, showing that having these programs and policies in place in general can cause general improvements in nutritional decision-making for children. However, the other frequent behavior changes at each site show the direct effects of the programs in place. In Palau, the other most commonly cited change in behavior was willingly eating more fruits and vegetables. At VES, it was assisting with cooking at home that garnered the most frequent responses from participants. This data is representative of the influence that programs can have on specific behaviors; in Palau, the Healthy Snacks policy that requires children to bring fruits and vegetables to school positively influences their choices to consume these items more often. In Southwest Virginia, the programs in place consist largely of cooking demonstrations and lessons; thus the tendency for children to practice more cooking with parents at home.

Students are, in fact, learning about healthy eating and developing better nutrition habits in school. The perspectives of these various stakeholders involved, however, clearly influence the specific programs and policies that are created, implemented, and sustained in schools. Therefore, carrying over these new ideas and behaviors into the home is crucial: if parents and other family members are not aware or supportive of the nutrition education efforts going on in their child's school, it makes it exceptionally difficult to see real behavior change that carries over at home and becomes long-term lifestyle change in students. Similarly, parent buy-in and parents helping their children make healthier choices could improve health outcomes for the whole family. Therefore, investigating parent involvement is a crucial part of school nutrition programming.

Parents' Perceptions of Program and Policy Success

Another important area of exploration was an investigation of parent attitudes toward the Healthy Snacks and H_2O Only policies in place at KES, and the activities and programs at VES. At the study site in Palau, policies in place only allow children to bring healthy snacks (fruits and vegetables) and water to class. At VES, programs in place focus primarily on hosting cooking demonstrations and teaching children how to eat and prepare fresh foods. School gardening is present at both sites, as well; parents and students are both involved with the school garden in Palau, while the garden program in Virginia is less popular for students and parents alike: very few parents indicated that their children had participated in the garden program, and no parents indicated being involved themselves. Variables measured included level of satisfaction with the policy or program, challenges associated with enforcing the policies, as well as ways the policies could be improved or changed.

The vast majority (75%) of parents at KES were in agreement that the Healthy Snacks policy was "somewhat" or "very successful." Meanwhile, parents believed the H_2O Only policy to be even more successful, with nearly all parents (90%) expressing approval. Parents who felt that the Healthy Snacks policy was successful reported decreased consumption of junk food and healthier choices being made by their children as the key positive outcomes of the policy, writing "my son does not ask for junk food anymore," and, "he is choosing more healthy foods." Many parents shared their own problems with enforcement, however. "I need to continuously encourage my child the importance of water. Also, with her peer group, they tend to drink sweets," wrote one parent, and many other parents said they experienced the same challenges with the H_2O Only policy. Discussion of the Healthy Snacks policy contained many of the same issues: "I still see children bringing unhealthy snacks to school," wrote one parent. "Healthy fruits are kind of expensive," wrote another. The issue of consistency both at home and at school was present here as well. One parent described it best by saying, "at home she can eat whatever she likes to eat." At VES, when asked how successful parents felt these programs were in improving their family's overall knowledge of nutrition, about half of parents (56%) felt these programs were either "somewhat" or "very successful."

In terms of the foods served at each school, about a quarter of parents in Palau were "very unsatisfied" or "unsatisfied" with the nutritional value of the foods served at school. Parents at KES mentioned improving school food as the main idea for improvement of school programs and polices in general. "Maybe school should charge (on a sliding scale) for lunch so more nutritional lunches can be provided instead of hot dogs, can food," said one parent. "School has to invest in healthy food. Charge parents if they have to as long as they get healthy food," wrote another.

At VES, slightly fewer parents were "very unsatisfied" or "unsatisfied" with school foods, while more than half of parents were "satisfied" or "very satisfied." Parents here, too, cited changes or improvements in school foods served most often when asked for their general ideas. "All schools should provide healthy lunches," wrote one parent. "Making sure that the school lunches are better quality," wrote another. Parents also talked about healthier school breakfasts, a meal that many students at the VES study site depend on. "The breakfast looks like a lot of sugary cereals," and "the food choice for breakfast could be a little more healthy," were two of the responses.

On the whole, parents seemed less satisfied with the foods served at school in Palau, but a significant number of parents at both study sites showed a certain level of disapproval, creating opportunities for change. At VES, 93% of students qualify for free lunch (National Center for Education Statistics 2012). In Palau, school lunch is always free for students, but constrained by financial challenges and a national policy that requires each school to serve the same foods in every school across the country (thus limiting the nutritional quality of the foods served). Here, too, we see the influence of different forms of community partnerships play out in the efficacy of programs and policies.

The Importance of Parent Involvement

Parent involvement and perceived success of programs/overall satisfaction were closely related. The extent to which parents were involved in the nutrition programs at each study site was perhaps one of the most obvious differences. While about half of parents at the site in Palau said that they had been involved with activities at their child's school to some extent, only one parent expressed involvement with nutrition-related programs and activities at their child's school in Southwest Virginia.

Parent involvement is a crucial element in carrying healthy eating messages through from school to the home. At KES, teachers confirmed that many parents were involved in nutrition programs and activities at school over the past year. They also emphasized the importance of parent involvement for long-term behavior change, writing about challenges with what students are learning not being enforced at home. "Getting the message across is the easy part, it's the implementation that's difficult. When students are in school their diet is more controlled, it's when they go home that they're exposed to unhealthy eating habits," explained one teacher.

Parents who were involved said that they enjoyed spending time with their children, and believed it was very good for their child's overall health to be involved, but they also expressed many barriers to involvement. Time to commit to participating in these programs is often scarce as parents balance multiple jobs and children. "Sometimes the program falls during work and my wife and I have to decide who should come because we are both working," one parent noted. "I have to take off or break at work because I work 7 days," said another Palauan parent. Parents at VES mirrored this as well: "I wish they did the program more than once a week so I could be involved." Parents mentioned other time constraints, like childcare for younger children, as a barrier as well. These barriers are mirrored by current literature on parent involvement at their children's schools in the United States, particularly when it comes to nutrition- related activities (Lamb-Parker et al. 2001; Hornby and Lafaele 2011). Finding ways to mitigate these seemingly cross-cultural barriers to parent involvement is an important area for research and program design, and the model by which programs are designed and implemented may be one way to address these barriers.

Models of Community-Based Intervention in Schools

Parental involvement and coalition stakeholder influence in the school-based interventions at KES and VES clearly differ. A key source of that difference may well lie in who drives the decision making process. At VES the model used is a community health coalition-based model. In the United States, the "coalition," defined by Feighery and Rogers as "an organization of individuals representing diverse organizations, factions or constituencies who agree to work together in order to achieve a common goal," often plays a major role in the development, implementation, and funding of programs. The coalition model for community change has become increasingly popular, and for good reason. Coalitions are often grant or federal program-driven and rely on an emphasis of partnerships between various community stakeholders, and thus provide a key access point for community members, marginalized groups, and grassroots leaders to create positive and sustainable changes within a community, particularly when they are given the opportunity to create connections with coalition members from powerful institutions (Everett 2011).

In Palau, decisions about school policies and programs surrounding nutrition are made by school officials themselves, with significant input from the Parent-Teacher Association (PTA). The PTA has a high attendance rate, with a majority of parents attending each meeting. It is through this extensive communication between parents, teachers, and school officials that ideas are formed and programs and policies are implemented. In the Republic of Palau, where changes are largely driven by the PTA and local administrators it is possible that there is a different level of buy-in in place, and thus, we may see differences in levels of success and parent attitudes than coalition-driven approaches. Even with high levels of involvement, there are challenges in maintaining parent support and in parents' buy-in at home.

At VES, there are significantly lower rates of parent participation and involvement in programming. The role of the coalition is a key factor here. The coalition serves as an holistic approach to health improvement, as it seeks to look beyond individual behaviors and risk factors and shifts the focus to improving health outcomes for an entire community (Everett 2011). However, an emphasis on singular levels of health (organizational, public policy, interpersonal) by coalitions often results in an oversight that reduces the effectiveness of the coalition's work—neglecting to gain the perspective of "members of the community groups that coalitions themselves purport to represent" (Morris and Luque 2011, 4) by neglecting to include the parents of the children they aim to serve. Importantly, including parents in the planning and design phases of programs and policies may serve to mitigate many of the common barriers parents in this case study mentioned, and may also help them be better equipped to reinforce behaviors at home.

LESSONS LEARNED FROM A COMPARATIVE CASE STUDY

This type of health intervention outcome study confirms the importance of an applied anthropological approach. This is a departure from many of the more biomedical or public health-based approaches common in many of the studies mentioned above that are often used in implementing programs in schools but "fundamentally ignores the multiple school-level variables that may affect intervention effectiveness (such as financial concerns, labor issues, staff behavior, parental reactions, etc.)" (Coleman et al. 2012, 81). In comparing and contrasting these models of community involvement and their influence on school nutrition programming, it seems clear that leadership, resources, and parent involvement can all play a role. These factors differ quite significantly between the two study sites. Coleman and colleagues posit four major shortcomings that can account for the lack of success of programs in schools: (1) inability to change certain aspects of the school nutrition environment; (2) inability to restrict unhealthy foods brought to school from home; (3) "lack of integration of the intervention into daily school practice because of delivery by research staff"; and (4) problems implementing curriculum alongside the necessary curriculum for standardized testing (2012, 91). Stakeholder influence and questions of who is driving the programming at schools plays a key role in mitigating several of these shortcomings. Parent-driven approaches are better suited to establish consistency in efforts between home and school and can assist with approaches that integrate research findings into programs that parents can be a part of, support, and even organize themselves. Coalition-driven approaches tend to have access to more political and financial resources to change school nutrition environments and demand more policy changes while helping teachers navigate barriers related to time and resources.

The importance of a parent-driven approach to school nutrition interventions lies in several of its key components: recognizing the importance of a whole community as an identity, not just as a physical location; building on the strengths that are already present in the community; utilizing a thorough understanding of all stakeholders involved; and facilitating a collaborative approach of all of these stakeholders in all phases of research, program design and implementation, and follow up. Our data support the notion that widespread integration, in-home nutritional behavior change, and perceived program success are better supported by schools in which parents and teachers, as key stakeholders, play a significant role in program design and implementation. Again, this is not to say that the programs at the Virginia study site are not beneficial, but that their benefit could be heightened by greater reliance on stakeholder voices. Similarly, the Palau efforts could be improved were the schools better able to affect change at a policy level—something the coalition driving programming is perhaps better positioned to accomplish.

Specific lessons learned from KES's parent- and teacher-focused approach might include expanding school gardening programs with increased opportunities for parents to volunteer, and involving parents more directly in the scheduling and timing of programs, as well as the planning and design of the program itself. Offering programs at a variety of times (during school, after school, weekends and evenings) would allow more parents to participate, thus increasing the possibility for crucial carryover of good nutrition habits and ideas into the home. Developing stronger relationships between parents at schools (like KES has begun to do with its strong PTA involvement) can also help with the stronger sense of parent buy-in and influence, as well as creating a support network to help parents with ideas, overcoming challenges, and discussing how to better incorporate lessons their children learn from these programs at school into their home life. Another possible recommendation is to call for the further development of the U.S.' farm-to-school programs, and designing similar policies in Palau (and other countries). Using elements of VES' coalition model, a group of business and policy leaders (working closely alongside the PTA and school officials) could help create policy change and improve food offerings for KES and other schools throughout the country.

This particular comparative case study shows how cultural and political differences can result in different approaches to childhood obesity prevention and intervention efforts. However, this could serve as a springboard for other researchers who want to look to school-based approaches to nutrition education. Teachers often face the same barriers (lack of time, knowledge, and resources) to incorporating more discussion of healthy eating or implementing the nutrition-based curriculum they are being handed. Parents, too, tend to express the same difficulties (lack of time, cost, feeling uninformed) in getting involved with programs at their child's school or knowing how to continue those efforts at home. Here, we have two different approaches that seek to deal with these barriers in several different ways, providing future researchers with many ideas and areas that can be changed and improved upon in many other countries and communities.

Further, this research has emphasized the value of cross-cultural comparison of nutrition programs at a variety of different schools. In essence, the very presence of a point of comparison between the two schools provides a way for us to better understand the current state of program efficacy and assets and barriers of efforts at both schools more effectively. Having a point of comparison to look at how two different cultures approach the same problem with seemingly similar solutions, but with varied outcomes, highlights the subtle but key differences in the two approaches. Thus, we are able to make recommendations and draw conclusions that can better serve both of these study sites, and provide a better look into more generalizable and applicable understandings of school nutrition education around the world.

NOTE

1. I would like to thank Dr. Chad T. Morris, who served as faculty advisor on all phases of this research and was invaluable in data collection, analysis, and the many phases of writing that followed. I would also like to thank Dr. Elizabeth Ackley for her guidance and assistance with the Virginia phase of this project and allowing me access to the study site, as well as Dr. Shannon Anderson and Dr. Srikanth Mallavarapu who served on the committee under which this research was conducted and provided helpful feedback and advice.

Chapter 7

Addressing Obesity and Associated Medical Conditions in Latino Immigrant Communities in Southeast Georgia[1]

John S. Luque, Moya L. Alfonso, and Yelena N. Tarasenko

According to medical authorities and the popular press, the United States is in the midst of an "obesity crisis" with two-thirds of the adult population being obese or overweight (BMI ≥ 25) and one in every three adults being classified as obese (BMI ≥ 30) (An 2014). Obesity is of great public health concern because it is tied to higher rates of a number of chronic diseases, including type 2 diabetes, hypertension, coronary heart disease, and certain cancers (Apovian 2013). For example, rates of diabetes among Latinos are almost double those of non-Latino whites, and approximately 3.2 million Latinos in the United States have type 2 diabetes (Schiller et al. 2012). There are also significant medical costs associated with rising obesity rates, estimated at $147 billion per year in 2008, which amounts to almost 10% of all medical spending (Finkelstein et al. 2009).

Public health reports have identified Latinos as one of the demographic groups disproportionately affected by the obesity crisis due to the group's rapid population growth (Singh et al. 2011). Cultural factors such as equating prosperity with being overweight and providing treats to children as a gesture of affection have been cited as contributing factors to obesity in Latino populations (Freedman et al. 2011). Latinos have a higher prevalence of obesity approximately 39% of the adult Latino population is obese, compared to approximately 35% of the general U.S. population (Flegal et al. 2012). Obesity among immigrant Latinos in the United States has been attributed to dietary changes that occur as part of the acculturation process (New et al. 2013; O'Brien et al. 2014). In particular, Mexican American women have exhibited a statistically significant increase in obesity rates compared to other groups (Flegal et al. 2012). However, since the majority of Latinos in the United States are of Mexican origin, there is also a close connection to the public health situation in Mexico, which is experiencing its own obesity epidemic with adult obesity rates surpassing the rates in the United States (Elder 2013; Ro and Fleischer 2014). A review of systematic reviews on acculturation, nutrition, diabetes, and health disparities in Latinos has found that while there is evidence that acculturation is associated with poor dietary quality and obesity, there was no clear association between type 2 diabetes and acculturation (Perez-Escamilla 2011).

According to NHANES data, the adoption of unhealthy lifestyles and sedentary behavior, in particular by Mexican immigrants, is associated with negative health outcomes (Murillo et al. 2014). In a study of acculturation and diabetes prevalence using NHANES data, higher acculturation levels were associated with an increased likelihood of diabetes, suggesting possible bio-behavioral mechanisms affecting dietary choices (O'Brien et al. 2014). Researchers at the Centers for Disease Control and Prevention (CDC) have examined particular dietary practices such as consumption of sugar-sweetened beverages. Using BRFSS data, they analyzed rates of consumption by race and ethnicity to identify differences among groups and found a higher intake in non-Latino blacks and Latinos than in other ethnic groups (Kumar et al. 2014). While the aforementioned studies focused on individual characteristics, structural factors such as food marketing are also connected to behavioral changes in dietary practices. Although some researchers might interpret snack food and sugar-sweetened beverage marketing in the United States as the major driver for changing consumption patterns of Latino immigrants, there is a long history of so-called "coca-colonization" to market "calorie-dense but nutrient-poor" foods to diverse ethnic groups in Mexico (Leatherman and Goodman 2005).

There exist health disparities between non-Latino whites and Latinos with type 2 diabetes (Perez-Escamilla 2011). The prevalence rate of diabetes for Latinos is 13.2%, which is 70% higher than the rate for non-Latino whites (Schiller et al. 2012). One region of the U.S. which has particularly been affected by the obesity crisis and associated health conditions is the southeastern United States. A wave of Latino immigrants, primarily from Mexico, arrived in the region beginning in the 1990s to work in agriculture and industrial food production (Griffith 2005). The demographic picture of the southeastern U.S. is changing, as states such as North Carolina, South Carolina, and Georgia have experienced rapid population growth of their Latino populations over the last two decades. Between 2000 and 2010, the U.S. South was characterized by a 57% increase in its Latino population; during which time the total U.S. population increased by only 14% (Ennis et al. 2011).

The southeastern U.S. has the highest rates of obesity in the country, caused by a confluence of factors along the socioecologic spectrum (Maddock 2004). Recent studies focused on Latino childhood obesity have taken an ecological approach and focused on structural factors, such as food deserts, lack of exercise opportunities, and food marketing as major factors contributing to the problem (Ramirez et al. 2013). There have been relatively few intervention studies in the southeastern United States to reduce obesity among Latinos. In a qualitative study conducted in Alabama, researchers found Latina women attributed depression, social isolation, and a lack of social support to weight gain and stressed the importance of family involvement in weight-loss programs (Agne et al. 2012). In rural areas of Georgia, obesity and associated diseases also affect Latino immigrants. A recent study of Latino farmworker children in southwestern Georgia found an obesity prevalence ranging from 24% to 37% for an eight-year period. These prevalence estimates were significantly higher than those ranging from 13% to 22% based on NHANES data for a comparison group of Mexican American children (Nichols et al. 2014).

In strictly biological terms, excess weight and high body mass index (BMI) are correlated with the rising incidence of type 2 diabetes. Individuals who do not produce sufficient insulin secretion to align with insulin resistance will not be able to maintain normal glucose tolerance (Al-Goblan et al. 2014). This in turn may lead to the development of diabetes in individuals with a high BMI.

Given the growing problem of obesity and obesity-related diseases for the Latino population, investigators have developed interventions both in Latin America and in the United States and evaluated them for their effectiveness in curbing obesity (Holub et al. 2013). Most obesity-related interventions entail individual and behavioral modifications to eat healthier and exercise more. These individual-centered approaches have been critiqued by proponents of the significance of structural factors for curbing obesity in Latino populations (Greenhalgh and Carney 2014).

Several recent systematic reviews have documented interventions for combating the obesity crisis among Latinos. Holub et al. (2013) reviewed 105 intervention studies, with over half conducted in the United States. The review divided the studies based on whether the interventions targeted adults or children, and by geographical region. Six studies provided strong evidence for individual-based interventions to improve physical activity and healthy eating aimed at either overweight or obese U.S. Latino adults with an average effect size of obesity-related measures (i.e., BMI and weight) of .30. These intervention studies consisted of classes delivered in community locations, most commonly by a registered dietitian, and ranged in duration from two to six months. For Latino children, school-based interventions that combined physical activity with healthy eating were found to be the most effective when including parents, addressing the cultural importance of the family. In another review, which only examined treatment interventions targeting U.S. Latino obese adults, Perez et al. (2013) found that of the 22 studies identified, more than half suggested significant improvements for BMI and weight. However, few of the studies reported follow-up measurements, thus limiting conclusions on the long-term results of these interventions. One study used a factorial design to evaluate different components of a multi-level intervention targeted to Latino children and parents in southern California (Crespo et al. 2012). The study examined the effects of parenting and community environments to prevent childhood obesity in young Latino elementary school children. The results showed no combined effect of intervening on the two environments simultaneously, but did find that changes in parenting practices had a significant effect on the child's behaviors related to diet and physical activity. Greenhalgh and Carney (2014, 269) have argued that instead of individual-based interventions, what is really needed are more ethnographic studies to "disentangle the social, structural, and intergenerational dynamics of higher prevalence of overweight and obesity among United States-based Latino populations." Hopefully, these types of studies would result in identifying real-world solutions to intervene at multiple levels (i.e., targeting both the individual and the environment).

This chapter provides two examples of community-based interventions targeting Latino adults in rural southeast Georgia. The first intervention was community-driven, and the investigator was only involved in program evaluation efforts. There is substantial evidence that a large amount of useful public health information is not indexed in article databases, and is only accessible through reports from governmental and nonprofit organizations (Turner et al. 2005). This chapter disseminates the results of the program evaluation. The intervention utilized a non-medical case-management approach to serve Latino patients with type 2 diabetes. The section describes the results of intervention and evaluation data analyses suggesting behavioral changes in the Latino clients served. The second intervention was investigator-driven and served as the control condition in a community efficacy trial targeting Latina immigrant women to receive up-to-date cervical cancer screening. In many intervention studies, the effects on control condition participants are underreported and only discussed in terms of differences with the primary variables of interest for the intervention arm. There are fewer studies which explore changes in participants in the control arm for active control conditions; moreover, the selection of the control condition can have an impact on the outcomes of efficacy trials, such as greater difficulty in detecting treatment effects using active comparison conditions (Freedland et al. 2011; Mohr et al. 2009). The section describes a nutrition workshop intervention that was delivered to Latina immigrant women and presents preliminary evaluation data from baseline surveys.

EVALUATION OF A COMMUNITY-BASED DIABETES INTERVENTION

Applied anthropologists and evaluators are often contacted to conduct evaluations of community-based interventions. This section provides a case study of one such evaluation. In 2012, one of the chapter authors (JL) was contracted to complete an outcome evaluation of two years of a diabetes self-management program titled *LaRED* (*Latinos Reduciendo el Diabetes*—Latinos Reducing Diabetes), delivered by a community-based organization, Southeast Georgia Communities Project (SEGCP) located in Lyons, Georgia. SEGCP serves to help their mostly Latino clients with translation services, health education, and assistance with communicating with health and social services providers. SEGCP is managed by two Mexican American sisters, whose parents were farmworkers in Texas and the southeastern U.S. There is a history of collaboration between SEGCP and the Georgia Southern University Jiann-Ping Hsu College of Public Health including program evaluation efforts, collaboration on annual migrant farm clinics and *promotora* training initiatives focused on cervical cancer education (Luque et al. 2011, 2012; Mason 2009).

Diabetes Intervention Description

Recognizing that the problem of diabetes was very prevalent in the Mexican immigrant farmworker community, SEGCP received funding from both the Health Resources and Services Administration (HRSA) and later the Healthcare Georgia Foundation to implement the CDC's *Take Charge of Your Diabetes* program (Centers for Disease Control and Prevention 2007), a diabetes self-management program. The goal of this program was to reduce diabetes-related morbidity and mortality by providing culturally and linguistically appropriate non-medical case management, education and support services to adult Latino diabetic clients residing in a seven-county area of rural southeast Georgia (Appling, Candler, Emanuel, Evans, Long, Tattnall, Toombs). The two primary methods utilized by SEGCP to reach their goal were to provide: (1) education and non-medical case management during home visits by trained bilingual diabetes prevention and management advocates, and (2) healthy lifestyle and diabetes prevention education to adults and youth in one-on-one sessions, group settings, and telephone counseling sessions.

Diabetic clients could receive testing supplies from SEGCP at a very low (or no) cost if they did not have the financial resources to obtain their own. Medication assistance was also provided through a sustainability plan in partnership with a private company that produces glucometers. The private company provided the glucometers free of cost when testing strips were ordered. SEGCP purchased testing strips for \$.40 per strip, which was more affordable than the \$1.50 most clients paid at most pharmacies or doctor's offices. SEGCP requested a client donation of \$20 for a box of 50 strips. However, if the client was unable to afford to pay for the strips, they were provided at no cost. SEGCP also assisted with medication purchases for clients in some cases, when clients were unable to travel to the pharmacy. SEGCP outreach workers purchased the medications and delivered them to the client's home. The funds received from clients for testing strips enabled SEGCP to purchase more strips and to provide supplies to those who could not afford them.

As part of their regular day-to-day activities, SEGCP provided bilingual services for non-English-speaking clients in surrounding counties for agencies such as the Department of Family and Child Services, a regional Community Health Center, local hospitals, and local merchants. Most of the diabetes client referrals were made to the Community Health Center, and nurses from that organization reported that the diabetic clients referred by SEGCP were compliant patients. Based on a 2009 evaluation report, there was minimal attrition over a two-year period for the 138 Latino diabetic clients enrolled in the program (56% female, 41% male). The report stated that five clients moved out of the area. Moreover, there were positive self-reported dietary behavior changes such as eating more fruits and vegetables and drinking more water (and less sugar-sweetened beverages). In addition, clients reported taking their medications, checking blood glucose levels, and having their A1C checked. Fifty-three of these clients received supplies for diabetes self-management (glucometers and test strips). The average baseline readings of the 99 clients who had their blood glucose levels tested with A1C checked 9.3% for the baseline and 8.7% for the follow-up readings with 72 clients. The values showed promise for the program with 58% of clients demonstrating reduced A1C levels (Mason 2009).

Diabetes Intervention Evaluation Findings

For the subsequent 2012 evaluation report, which covered the years from 2010 to 2011, there were 134 Latino diabetic clients served by the *LaRED* program. Because the evaluator did not have access to the 2009 database, it could not be determined how many of the same clients continued with the program from the previous evaluation period (Luque 2012). Over 1,186 non-medical case management client encounters were provided by SEGCP program staff. The majority of encounters were home visits (63.4%) followed by outreach (15.9%), telephone calls (12.9%), case management (5.6%), and interpretation (2.1%). In the two-year timeframe, 128 female clients had their A1C levels measured longitudinally. The outcome evaluation concluded that participants who had started the program with an A1C level above the recommendation of the American Diabetes Association (>7% A1C), showed a statistically significant change of –1.87% A1C based on a paired *t*-test [–2.35%, –1.38%] ($p < 0.001$). Participants with higher pre-test A1C levels also experienced larger decreases in A1C levels during the program.

In addition to A1C levels, the program measured lifestyle factors. Twelve diabetes prevention workshops were held over the two-year period and attended by 15 to 43 participants per workshop for a total of 100 participants. Forty-three clients received the first session of the education curriculum, which is a basic introduction to diabetes. Out of a maximum of 100%, the average pretest score of clients was 79% and the average posttest score was 97%. Out of all the sessions, 27% of participants had a pretest score of 100%, but 86% of participants had a posttest score of 100%. Table 7.1 reports mean pretest and posttest scores for each workshop. Based on paired *t*-tests, the score increases were all statistically significant at the $p < 0.05$ level. The largest score increases were observed with the sessions on Vaccinations (Session 11), Emotional & Eye Problems (Session 4 and 5), Keeping Track of your Glucose (Session 3), Nerve Damage (Session 8), and Controlling your Diabetes (Session 2). The overall average percentage increase for all the sessions was 21% (results not shown). The sequence of session delivery was based on the topics of interest that received priority in the conversations between staff and clients. Figure 7.1 displays the education session results. Overall, the behaviors that demonstrated the most improvements (from high to low frequency) included: (1) limiting alcohol intake; (2) taking medications regularly; (3) checking blood sugar daily; (4) drinking eight glasses of water per day; and (5) eating more fruit. The only lifestyle change that did not improve was exercising 30 minutes per day. The evaluation identified the following recommendations to improve the diabetes intervention for clients: (1) stressing the importance of the A1C test; (2) getting vision tests; (3) eating more vegetables; (4) getting feet checked; and (5) limiting salt intake. The SEGCP staff shared that they had to convince some clients of the importance of taking medications instead of ingesting natural remedies such as prickly pear cactus juice.

Because the majority of clients worked as farmworkers, their time was very limited, and the outreach services provided regular monitoring of dietary intake and medication usage that worked around their client's busy schedules. In the final year of the program (2012), which was not part of the evaluation report, 45 clients received outreach and non-medical case management, and there were a total of 209 encounters. Based on these data, clients continued to encounter challenges with having their vision and feet checked.

The results of the outcome evaluation of this community-based program demonstrated that non-medical case management of diabetes could produce very positive results using limited resources. The program employed culturally competent, bilingual staff to address the needs of their Latino clients. By focusing on home visits where the family was present to observe the interactions, the staff helped their clients both control their diabetes and modify their lifestyle to improve overall health. While this program did focus on individual behaviors through the workshop intervention approach, it also addressed structural factors, such as cost, by subsidizing reduced cost testing strips and by providing free medications to those facing transportation barriers.

Table 7.1 *LaRED* Education Workshop Session Data (2010–2011)

	Session[a]	*Mean Pretest*	*Mean Posttest*	*Mean Increase*	*p-value*
1	Introduction (N = 43)	79.8	96.7	16.9	<0.001
2	Controlling Diabetes (N = 29)	79.1	99.1	20.0	<0.001
3	Tracking Glucose (N = 26)	68.5	96.9	28.4	<0.001
4/5	Emotional & Eye Problems (N = 26)	67.0	98.5	31.5	<0.001
6	Kidney Problems (N = 36)	75.4	93.0	17.6	<0.001
7	Heart & Blood Vessels (N = 32)	86.9	95.3	8.4	0.025
8	Nerve Damage (N = 35)	72.4	97.1	24.7	<0.001
9	Foot Problems (N = 29)	76.1	94.1	18.0	<0.001
10	Dental Disease (N = 29)	79.7	96.4	16.7	<0.001
11	Vaccinations (N = 19)	59.7	95.6	35.9	<0.001
12	Pregnancy/Women's Health (N = 15)	87.3	100.0	12.7	<0.001

[a]Sessions are listed in order according to curriculum materials.

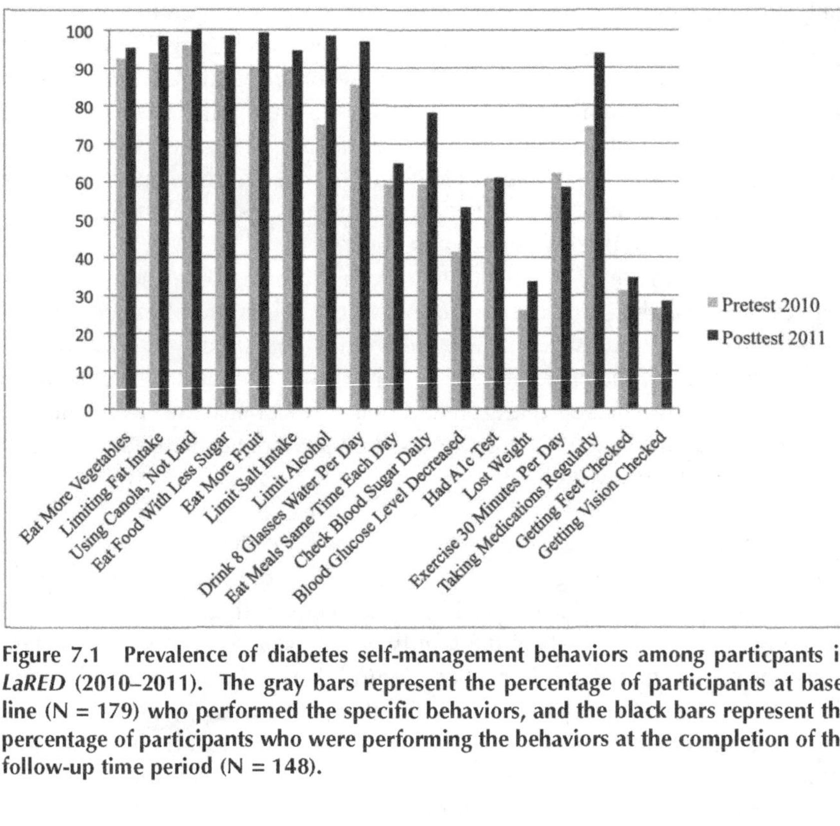

Figure 7.1 Prevalence of diabetes self-management behaviors among particpants in *LaRED* (2010–2011). The gray bars represent the percentage of participants at baseline (N = 179) who performed the specific behaviors, and the black bars represent the percentage of participants who were performing the behaviors at the completion of the follow-up time period (N = 148).

DEVELOPMENT OF A NUTRITION EDUCATION WORKSHOP INTERVENTION

The evaluation of the *LaRED* diabetes program described above informed the development of a nutrition workshop intervention delivered in a neighboring community with a similar Latino immigrant population (i.e., Mexican farmworkers), as part of a NIH-funded *promotora* (lay health advisor) intervention efficacy study on cervical cancer screening titled *Salud es Vida* (Health is Life). The study purpose was to test the efficacy of *promotoras,* or lay health advisors, to increase cervical cancer screening in underscreened Latina immigrant women. The nutrition workshop served as the control condition for the study. In close collaboration with community organizations and the faith community, nutrition workshops were delivered to small groups of Latina immigrant women.

Efficacy Trial Overview

The nutrition workshop employed multiple learning components (video, didactic presentation, and interactive activities). Latina women between the ages of 21 and 65 who were born outside of the U.S. and had not received a Pap test for over two years were eligible for the study. Participants were recruited from churches, schools, businesses, and community venues through posters, word-of-mouth and flyers. The intervention lasted from November 2013 to January 2015. A total of 19 workshops were held, enrolling 79 participants. Each workshop was led by the nutrition student/research assistant and was co-facilitated by the project coordinator. Workshop sessions were designed to be informative and interesting, thus, the emphasis was on active learning strategies, such as sampling healthy foods and reading nutrition labels.

Nutrition Education Workshop Description

A nutrition student/research assistant from Honduras and a project coordinator from Colombia led the creation of the nutrition education workshop structure, along with two of the chapter co-authors (MA, JL). At the foundation of the workshop was a 10-minute nutrition video titled *Nutrición: Alimentación Saludable* (Nutrition: Healthy Eating) (Clínica Naturista de Medicina Integral 2014). This video was selected because it was easy to understand, contained basic information about nutrition, was created for Spanish speakers, and was slow paced with engaging visuals. Once the video was selected, a PowerPoint presentation was developed to accompany the video. The PowerPoint presentation expanded on the basic nutrition information covered in the video and provided examples of types of foods that contained specific nutrients. In addition to the video and PowerPoint presentation, participants engaged in interactive activities including a nutrition label activity that taught participants how to interpret nutrition facts, a demonstration of simple, nutritious recipes, and examples of how to find healthy foods in the grocery store. A workshop session agenda is provided in Table 7.2.

The workshop began with an introduction followed by the video. The video highlighted the importance of a healthy lifestyle and a balanced diet, as well as some basic concepts about nutrition, such as the essential nutrients needed for a healthy diet as well as some types of food people should avoid. After the video, the workshop facilitator provided an interactive PowerPoint presentation based on the topics covered in the video. The presentation began with a detailed description of basic nutrients, their different sources, and why they were important for the body, for example, due to being content-rich in vitamins A, B (B1, B9, B12), C, D, E, K; in minerals (calcium, potassium, iron, zinc); fat (saturated and unsaturated); and in water. In addition to all the essential nutrients, participants were taught the basic aspects of processed and refined food—because they were not familiar with the terms—and how consumption of such foods could negatively affect a person's health. Whole grains were emphasized as a source of healthy carbohydrates in the diet. Different sources of proteins were mentioned in the video and the PowerPoint presentation to show the participants alternative non-animal sources of protein. Participants also learned about the different types of fat, to avoid

Table 7.2 Nutrition Workshop Agenda (two-hours duration)

Agenda Item	*Item Description*
Arrival	Participant completes sign-in sheet and child care arrangements are made.
Icebreaker	Participants engage in an icebreaker exercise prior to the lesson.
Evaluation	Participants receive informed consent and participate in the pretest survey.
Food preparation	The co-facilitator prepares the sample recipes of the day (e.g., pasta, salad, hummus, fruit smoothies, salad, water with lemon, cucumber and mint).
Nutrition Video	Participants watch the nutrition video – *Nutrición: Alimentación Saludable*.
Nutrition PowerPoint	Participants listen to the PowerPoint presentation from the facilitator and ask questions.
Hands On Activity	Participants engage in hands-on activities, including a nutrition label reading and interpretation exercise.
Break	Participants take a break and enjoy sample recipes.
Brochures	Participants receive educational brochures.
Evaluation	Participants take the posttest survey.

saturated fat, and how plant sources of fat, such as nuts, olives, and avocados, are important in the diet for absorption of fat-soluble vitamins. In contrast, reasons why saturated fats are unhealthy were discussed because some Latino families cook with animal fat. Finally, the presentation discussed how to make healthy food choices based on proportions of vegetables, proteins, fruits, and starches.

Anecdotally, participants reported they did not pay much attention to what was stated on the product labels of the foods they purchased; therefore, it was a surprise for them to find out about all of the relevant nutrition information they could obtain from these labels. They were particularly interested in learning more about the 5-20 Label Rule, which provides guidance for the recommended daily nutrient intakes (U.S. Food and Drug Administration 2015). The 5% applies to intake of saturated fats, trans fats, cholesterol, and sodium; whereas, the 20% applies to intake of nutrients such as fiber, vitamins A and C, calcium, and iron. To make the food-labeling workshop component more appealing, products often consumed by the participants and healthy options were presented as examples and product packages were used for the activity. The women especially enjoyed the nutrition label exercise and asked several questions.

Participants also showed interest in learning more about portion sizes. This topic was related to the nutrition facts label part of the presentation, since portion sizes play a role in determining the intake of nutrients. Participants were surprised to learn that for some foods, what they considered a normal portion size often exceeded what the label indicated as equal to one portion size. The women appreciated learning about reading nutrition facts labels so they could calculate portion sizes to feed their families and make healthier choices when buying food products. After the video, participants received handouts that contained a summary of the information that was covered during the session and provided guidelines and activities to learn how to read and interpret nutrition facts labels as well as learn healthy recipes.

Toward the end of the workshop, the participants sampled some of the healthy food recipes prepared for the session. These foods included a cucumber-lemon water beverage; vegetable whole grain pasta dish; fat-free hummus and pita bread; spinach salad topped with cranberries, nuts and "lite" raspberry vinaigrette dressing; and a fruit smoothie. According to the workshop facilitators, participants enjoyed the variety of foods that were new to them, as well as the ease of preparation and the nutritional value.

Evaluation Methods

All participants (intervention and control) completed a baseline survey, which included knowledge measures on healthy foods and attitudes toward food choices and meal preparation, in addition to the cervical cancer questions and demographic information. Knowledge (recall) posttest scores were collected immediately following each class. Baseline data were collected from 86 participants in the treatment condition (*promotora*-led cervical cancer education) and 90 participants in the control condition (nutrition workshop). Moreover, six-month follow-up surveys were collected from nutrition workshop participants. The average age of the nutrition workshop participants was 38 years old, with an average of 13 years living in the United States. Approximately 82% of participants were born in Mexico, and the rest were mostly from Honduras or Guatemala.

Nutrition Education Workshop Findings

On a 14-question nutrition knowledge true/false test, the cervical cancer education group baseline and posttest mean scores were the same 11.5 (SD = 1.7, 1.5). In the nutrition workshop group, the mean posttest score of 11.9 (SD = 1.6) was higher than the mean baseline score of 11.5 (SD = 1.8), based on the Wilcoxon signed rank test ($p = 0.03$). Findings from the six-month follow-up surveys suggest this nutrition knowledge was retained with a mean score of 12.1 (SD = 1.3). In the posttest, the nutrition workshop participants still had difficulty with questions about whether a diet full of processed foods could produce cancer and whether fats were important for a healthy diet - both true statements. Item analysis suggested improved knowledge of nutrition workshop participants in the following areas: the relationship between processed foods and cholesterol, the importance of obtaining key vitamins and nutrients from whole foods (as opposed to multivitamins), and the dangers of consuming an excess of saturated fats for adults and children.

Participants also responded to 14 questions concerning their food consumption patterns in both the baseline and the follow-up surveys. These items included questions such as, "Do you eat 3 meals per day?" "Do you try not to eat too much?" and "Do you eat vegetables daily?" Response options were on a 3-point scale (1 = "no"; 2 = "sometimes"; and 3 = "yes"). For these questions, the average responses ranged between "sometimes" and "yes," indicating that participants leaned toward positive perceived healthy eating behaviors. These positive patterns continued with the follow-up surveys from our preliminary data. In particular, there was an inclination toward not eating foods cooked with oil at every meal. In addition, participants provided answers to questions about influences on their food preparation habits on a 5-point Likert scale (1= "strongly disagree" to 5 = "strongly agree") based on constructs from Social Cognitive Theory (self-efficacy, reciprocal determinism, self-regulation, and observational learning) on the baseline survey only (Bandura 2004). The average scores of these questions for the nutrition workshop participants are presented in Table 7.3. In the baseline survey for nutrition workshop participants, 81% either agreed or strongly agreed that their family determined what they ate, showing high reciprocal determinism. In addition, 83% either agreed or strongly agreed that they could prepare healthy foods, showing positive self-efficacy for the ability to eat healthy.

The evaluation of the control condition showed that this group exhibited a high level of interest in participating in the nutrition education workshops. Similar to the diabetes intervention described earlier, results from the nutrition workshops demonstrated that participants ate a more balanced diet, reduced their consumption of salty foods, and consumed more fruits and vegetables. This intervention was a group-based rather than an individual-based intervention, so it is possible that participants continued the discussion about

Table 7.3 Nutrition Survey Questions

Survey Item	*Mean Baseline Score*[c]	*SD*	*Mean Follow-Up Score*[d]	*SD*
Food Choices[a]				
Eat three meals daily	2.21	.67	2.25	.65
Eat foods slowly	2.01	.78	2.20	.75
Try not to eat/overeat	2.30	.78	2.52	.64
Try to eat a balanced diet	2.16	.82	2.59	.61
Try not to eat salty foods	2.25	.82	2.49	.73
Eat rice, bread, pasta, or tortillas at every meal	2.23	.78	2.37	.82
Eat meat, eggs, fish, beans daily	2.16	.69	2.40	.75
Eat foods cooked with oil at every meal	2.10	.75	1.94	.77
Eat milk, cheese, cream, butter daily	2.19	.75	2.17	.76
Eat vegetables daily	2.07	.68	2.61	.53
Eat fruits daily	2.28	.73	2.47	.64
Enjoy your food	2.64	.61	2.92	.27
Individual, Social, and Environmental Influences on Food Habits[b]				
What my family eats is what I eat	4.02	1.13		
What I eat is what my family eats	4.10	1.09		
I can prepare healthy foods	4.21	0.93		
I know how to prepare healthy food for my family	3.68	1.22		
My friends teach me how to prepare healthy food	2.69	1.31		
I learned how to prepare healthy food on TV	2.74	1.26		
I learned how to prepare healthy food in this workshop	3.43	1.07		
I know what I should eat	3.78	1.22		
I choose to eat a healthy diet most of the time	3.58	1.22		

[a]Scale ranging from 1 to 3 (1 = "no", 2 = "sometimes", 3 = "yes")
[b]Likert scale ranging from 1 to 5 (1 = "strongly disagree", 2 = "disagree", 3 = "neutral", 4 = "agree", and 5 = "strongly agree")
[c]N = 90, baseline control group participants
[d]N = 52, only including follow-up surveys for participants who meet same inclusion criteria as cervical cancer education intervention group (e.g., not up-to-date with Pap test).

healthy cooking and eating after their exposure to the brief intervention. In both examples, a community group-based intervention approach toward obesity prevention was well received by participants.

CONCLUSIONS AND RECOMMENDATIONS

Applied anthropological approaches to evaluation and intervention development can contribute to efforts to target obesity intervention programs to Latino participants. In the first example, Latina staff at SEGCP delivered a CDC intervention to their Latino clients and engaged outsiders (applied anthropologists) to evaluate their efforts based on the project's stated aims and goals. The evaluator was able to review the data collected by program staff, interview all SEGCP staff involved with the program, and communicate with the health care manager at the area Community Health Center. Taken together, the evaluation data collected by two different evaluators concluded that the nonmedical case management approach to diabetes self-management for Latinos in this community was very effective, largely due to the exemplary efforts of SEGCP's staff and outreach workers to monitor their clients' needs. Unfortunately, given the short time period available to complete the outcome evaluation report, the evaluator was not able to interview *LaRED* clients served by the program, so this was one limitation of the evaluation. Nevertheless the client data showed several positive outcomes in terms of dietary changes, monitoring of blood glucose, and medication adherence.

Oftentimes, these types of community driven interventions are not published in the academic literature and are only available in the grey literature as project reports to funding agencies. Researchers and evaluators should work with community agencies to publish intervention findings so practitioners can better judge which programs adapt well to different settings and to other populations, as in this case with rural Latino immigrants. In addition, strategies to increase usability of evaluations should be integrated into the design. For example, through including stakeholders in the evaluation design, we were able to incorporate their feedback into the evaluation design, thereby increasing ultimate usability (Patton 1997). A key component of increasing usability is a focus on dissemination of evaluation results. In addition to peer-reviewed publications and white papers, additional efforts should be made to share evaluation findings with key stakeholders and communities seeking to implement similar programs (Patton 1997). Communities have much to learn from one another, and through sharing lessons learned, can improve interventions prior to implementation. Some lessons learned from this evaluation are that by including peer outreach workers in intervention delivery, being flexible with outreach contact (e.g., both home visits and telephone contacts) and providing low-cost medical supplies, the program was able to reach a larger number of individuals and effect positive change in clients with diabetes.

In the second example, our study team developed a nutrition education workshop targeted to Mexican immigrant women, identified in the literature as having higher obesity rates than some other groups (Flegal et al. 2012). Although our curriculum produced only modest changes in nutrition knowledge from pretest to posttest, item analysis suggested more nutrition vocabulary education was needed due to low education levels of our participants. Terms such as saturated, refined, processed, and whole grains were difficult for participants to understand and remember. Moreover, more education is needed about limiting processed, saturated fat and high sodium foods in the diet. Cultural influences were identified in some of the survey questions. For example, family influence is an important factor influencing dietary choices among Latinos (Gerchow et al. 2014; Greaney et al. 2012). Participants seemed to believe in a strong family effect on what they consumed and a weaker (or lesser) effect of friends on food preparation. Perhaps inviting entire families to participate in nutrition workshops rather than only adult women would produce better outcomes for nutrition interventions targeting Latino populations. Given the current popularity of food networks and shows on television, there was an item about whether women learned healthy cooking from television. Results showed that this was not perceived as influential among participants. However, participants were more positive in their responses that they learned about healthy cooking in the workshop. The results of the follow-up surveys suggested that knowledge was retained from the brief intervention.

A limitation of the second intervention should be considered—this active control condition for the two-arm efficacy study was developed by the study team without qualitative input from the target audience. Lindber, Stevens, and Halperin (2013) recommend the use of qualitative formative research when developing interventions for Latino populations given the diversity within this group. Future efforts to improve the nutrition intervention should include a series of focus group discussions with the target audience, with emphasis on exploring cultural and structural factors that should be included in the intervention. For example, participants could respond to questions about including family members in the intervention and strategies that would be effective in educating their peers on key nutrients, including healthy fats. Key components of the existing intervention could be tested for their cultural appropriateness and perceived effectiveness. Qualitative insights are needed prior to a subsequent intervention implementation. The feedback received during the one-on-one follow up surveys was very positive. Women expressed that they enjoyed the nutrition workshop and started to make some gradual changes in their daily food consumption, such as adding more fruits and vegetables, and consuming fewer "bad" fats. They also expressed a desire to attend more educational events if they became available.

Overall, the findings from these obesity-related interventions suggest that including bilingual/bicultural staff in intervention delivery, developing and evaluating programs in partnership with stakeholders, and sharing program findings with the community are all best practices in an applied context when collaborating with Latino communities. As the introduction to this chapter discussed, however, more studies are needed to measure longitudinal changes from these programs in diet, weight, and physical activity. In addition, multilevel interventions that work on the individual and environmental levels are required to maximize the potential for successful healthy nutrition and chronic disease self-management programs.

Applied anthropological research methods such as ethnography can provide rich contextual information to inform culturally appropriate interventions. While this chapter has discussed primarily public health approaches such as peer outreach and educational workshops, any national intervention strategy for Latinos needs to incorporate culturally competent approaches that resonate with target populations. Studies continue to provide evidence for the merit of public health approaches which emphasize that there will be greater gains from modifying unhealthy lifestyles and changing the obesogenic environment than taking the approach of biomedicine, which endeavors to better treat obesity-related conditions with the development of new medical procedures and medications.

NOTE

1. This work was supported by the National Cancer Institute, Office of the Director, under Grant Number R21 CA163159 and the Healthcare Georgia Foundation. The content is solely the responsibility of the authors and does not necessarily represent the official views of the National Cancer Institute or the National Institutes of Health. We acknowledge the assistance of Claudia Reyes-Garcia, Laura Rebing Amador, and Lisa Watson with developing the nutrition workshop intervention. We also acknowledge the collaboration of the Southeast Georgia Communities Project staff and leadership (Andrea Hinojosa, Director) on the *LaRED* program evaluation.

Chapter 8

Working with Low-Income and Latino Farmers to Increase Access to Oregon's Local Food Markets using Community Based Participatory Research and Public Participation GIS

Margaret Everett, Betty Izumi, Scott Ellis, Alejandro Tecum, Anne Morse, and Stacey Sobell

Though seemingly paradoxical, the relationship between hunger, obesity, and poverty is now well established in the public health literature. While obesity may commonly be viewed as "overconsumption," rates of food insecurity have grown alongside obesity rates in the United States. Ever since Dietz (1995) posited a causal relationship between hunger and obesity, researchers have sought to understand in detail the interactions between poverty, food access, diet quality, and health outcomes (Dinour et al. 2007; Drewnowski 2004, 2009; Adams 2003). This research demonstrated that obesity and food insecurity are both correlated to diet quality and food access with complex social, behavioral and environmental causes.

This chapter provides a case study of a Community-Based Participatory Research (CBPR)/Public Participation Geographic Information Systems (PPGIS) project that focused on the health concern of food insecurity for low-income populations. The study highlights the use of PPGIS as a technique to support a bottom-up participatory approach in order to diversify conversation points regarding the health issue at hand. Focused in the Oregon cities of Forest Grove and Cornelius, the project aimed at increasing access to local and regional economic markets for low-income Latino farmers in order to improve local consumer access to healthy foods. Despite a flourishing local food system in Oregon, food access varies significantly by income and ethnicity in the region, and low-income and Hispanic residents have significantly higher rates of obesity (Breyer and Voss-Andreae 2013; Oregon Health Authority 2012, 11). This community-university partnership sought to improve the access of Latinos to this local and sustainable food system as both consumers and producers in order to improve both health and economic disparities.

The project was funded by grants from the Northwest Health Foundation and the U.S. Department of Agriculture (USDA). Working with our community partners, Portland State University faculty and students provided evaluation and market research in support of the project. Project outcomes include detailed market analysis of local buyers and producers, increased access of low-income Latino farmers to local food markets, and increased supply of fresh, local produce available to low-income consumers. The project also enhanced the cultural competency of partner organizations to work with Latino and low-income farmers, and improved awareness among community members of the important role of Latino farmers.

Adelante Mujeres, a community organization serving Latina women and their families in Forest Grove, Oregon, served as the lead organization in the project. The organization's Sustainable Agriculture Program was created to empower and support Latinos as small-scale farmers and gardeners and to provide a market for their produce at the Forest Grove farmers market, which Adelante Mujeres operates. As Adelante Agricultura grew, farmers encountered market barriers that made it difficult to expand their businesses beyond the small farmers market. Adelante wanted to understand and address these barriers. PSU faculty and students provided evaluation and market research using a variety of methods, and partner organization Ecotrust provided market expertise and connections with institutional buyers in the region.

The academic partners in this project contributed tools and expertise from anthropology, public health and planning. Utilizing focus groups, interviews, surveys, and GIS they helped evaluate barriers and opportunities to build food security and expand market access for Latinos. Using Community-Based Participatory Research (CBPR) and Public Participation Geographic Information Systems (PPGIS), faculty and students supported a participatory approach that included a range of stakeholders.

BACKGROUND

The modern food system, consisting of heavily processed, fatty foods, has triggered a "nutrition transition" that has contributed to escalating rates of chronic disease and obesity (Popkin 2004). Nutritious foods such as fresh fruits and vegetables are more costly and less available in low-income areas; thus, low-income communities are particularly disadvantaged in such a system (Drewnowski 2004; Powell et al. 2007). In 2007, over 10 percent of Hispanics living in the United States had been diagnosed with diabetes

(Mainous et al. 2007).[1] The health risks associated with obesity, including heart disease, hypertension, and type 2 diabetes, are well-documented in the medical and public health literature. Oregon data on obesity rates reflect disparities by race and ethnicity. In Oregon, a 2007 report indicates that 70 percent of Hispanic adults are overweight or obese, compared to 60 percent of non-Hispanic whites (Nutrition Council of Oregon and the Oregon Coalition for Promoting Physical Activity 2007, 22). The same report notes that Hispanics in Oregon are less likely than whites to meet the USDA recommendation for daily fruit and vegetable intake.

Forest Grove and Cornelius have two of the fastest growing Hispanic populations in Oregon. According to the 2010 U.S. census, approximately 33 percent of the combined population of these towns is Hispanic. This is compared to the statewide average of 11.7 percent and the county average (Washington County) of 15.7 percent. Unfortunately, many of these Hispanic community members are impoverished. Approximately 24 percent of Latino residents in Washington County live under the poverty line (U.S. Census Bureau 2008).

Between 2010 and 2012, a community university partnership between Portland State University and two community organizations—Ecotrust and Adelante Mujeres—sought to address these issues in a rural community west of Portland, Oregon. The project focused on the Latino community of Washington County, where the lead organization, Adelante Mujeres, is located and has a strong community connection. Adelante Mujeres runs the Forest Grove Farmers market and runs several successful programs for Latinos in Forest Grove, but was interested in increasing promotion of the farmers market and in helping Latino farmers connect to local institutional buyers. The lead author reached out to Adelante Mujeres staff in 2009 regarding a funding proposal for an internal university sustainability grant. While that initial proposal was not funded, it led to discussions about how community-based research might help support Adelante's work. PSU faculty connected Adelante Mujeres to Ecotrust because of the organization's expertise in developing local sustainable food systems, and in 2010 the three organizations secured funding from a USDA Community Food Projects planning grant to improve market access for Latino farmers, with Adelante Mujeres serving as the lead organization. Also in 2010, the three organizations secured a two-year grant from the Northwest Health Foundation's grant program, "Preventing and Reducing Chronic Diseases through Policy Using Community Based Participatory Research." PSU supported the project by funding a Graduate Research Assistant, Scott Ellis, and funding the undergraduate survey research project.

Nationally, community food systems such as farmers markets and farm-to-school programs have the potential to narrow the gap between the food source (e.g., the farmer) and the consumer. These are identified as viable solutions to food insecurity and the resulting levels of chronic disease and obesity. Yet Latino community members and farmers are noticeably absent from this movement. Farm to school programs are one visible trend in the effort to improve market access for local farmers and improve dietary quality (for example, Story et al. 2008). The number of Latino-owned farms in Oregon increased by 11 percent between 2007 and 2012 (USDA 2012), but the project collaborators learned from community members that Latinos faced language, cultural, and economic barriers in their efforts to access local institutional markets such as farm to school programs. The same barriers may limit farmers market shopping among some Latino consumers. According to one study of farmers markets in low-income communities, these markets struggle to survive without subsidies, may not provide culturally desired foods, may lack sales staff with the same cultural and language background as the consumers, and may be difficult for low-income shoppers to access geographically (Fisher 1999). By researching ways to forge a stronger connection between producers and Latino consumers, we aimed to improve access to healthy foods by boosting participation in local food systems for low-income producers and consumers.

Project Partners

Adelante Mujeres, the lead community organization in this project, focuses on the development of grassroots, participatory approaches that are informed by the low-income Latino community. Through the practice of Paulo Freire's community education theory, Adelante Mujeres recognizes and embraces the benefits of co-learning and collaboration (Freire 2000). As an action-oriented community organization, Adelante Mujeres provided the research team and PSU students with the opportunity to pursue real world applications in a community setting. Adelante Mujeres staff helped recruit focus group participants, convened community meetings, and assisted with the implementation of a community assessment. As manager of the Forest Grove Farmers Market, Adelante Mujeres helped recruit participants for focus groups with vendors and with farmers, all led by PSU faculty and graduate students.

Ecotrust is an organization that works on broader conservation issues related to food and environmental justice on the Pacific Coast from Alaska to California. The role of Ecotrust in this project was to facilitate the partnership building process (e.g., through leading meetings and focus group sessions with Adelante Mujeres staff and program participants), relying on its organizational experience sharing knowledge and building community connections around sustainable food systems. Additionally, Ecotrust provided information on how to connect with institutional buyers in the region though its farm-to-school and Food Hub programs.

The partnership came together when the lead author reached out to Adelante for a letter of support on a grant proposal with PSU faculty to study whether and how Latino farmers have access to local food movement in northwest Oregon. While the initial proposal was not funded, it led to further discussions between Adelante Mujeres staff and PSU faculty about the need for improved market access for Latino and other low-income farmers in the region. At about this time, Ecotrust was launching its new Food Hub program, an online network designed to connect wholesale buyers and sellers within the northwest. While Ecotrust knew that Food Hub would greatly facilitate the growth of a local sustainable food system, they also knew that language and technology barriers could disadvantage low-income producers. When approached by PSU and Adelante Mujeres about applying for a U.S. Department of Agriculture Community Food Systems grant, they saw the potential to improve access to this new tool. Adelante Mujeres hoped the partnership would help increase the use of their farmers markets as well as assist farmers in identifying new institutional buyers beyond the farmers markets. For PSU faculty and students, the partnership presented a real world opportunity to study and address issues of food access and health inequalities.

Portland State University faculty in Community Health and Sociology worked with undergraduate students in a general education course and graduate students in urban planning to provide participatory research tools to guide the project. The PSU team guided the development of a mail survey, led focus groups, and conducted a GIS analysis of the survey results in order to facilitate community discussions on survey findings and next steps.

Rural Washington County

Adelante Mujeres developed an organic agriculture program in response to concerns about food security and chronic disease disparities among Latinos. The development of the Sustainable Agriculture program was an attempt to connect the surrounding low-income Latino community with more affordable, healthy food options. Specifically, this program provides aspiring Latino farmers with training as well as access to Adelante Mujeres' 12-acre farm to practice organic farming techniques. The program also provides training in business marketing along with space at the local Forest Grove Farmers Market to enable farmers to connect their products with local consumers. Adelante Mujeres created the farmers market to create opportunities for the farmers to sell their produce in the community. Ultimately, the goal of this program is to create a new source of affordable, healthy, and locally grown foods by helping local low-income Latino community members to start their own small scale farming operation and to connect their produce to local and regional markets. Workshops run for several weeks that provide both basic small-business training as well as agricultural know-how to help Latinos get started as small producers. Adelante Mujeres leased a 20 acre farm, which they named La Esperanza farm, and allowed those who had completed a workshop series to rent a small plot of land for a modest fee (water and some shared equipment were provided). Most farmers hold other jobs and families visit the farm in the evenings and weekends throughout the growing season to maintain their crops. The land was selected because of its relatively central location and its affordability.

After the inaugural harvest season of the Adelante Agricultura program in 2009, the participating community members and Adelante Mujeres staff concluded that the program lacked the information necessary for program success. Initial outreach efforts to promote the farmers market (posters and banners in the community announcing the market opening and an announcement inserted in the city's utility bill mailing each spring), had not generated enough traffic at the market for vendors to sell all of their produce. Moreover, farmers worried that they did not have enough understanding about what produce shoppers would purchase at the market. Adelante Mujeres did not possess a comprehensive understanding of the market barriers that farmers and consumers faced, nor did they have a strategic plan in place that outlined how they were to use their agriculture program to promote food security. This led to a Community Based Participatory Research (CBPR) project in order to better understand and address these questions. Between 2010 and 2012, the three project partners (PSU, Adelante Mujeres, Ecotrust) collaborated on three goals:

1. Assess the state of producer and consumer relationships among low-income and Latino farmers and low-income consumers.
2. Build the capacity and cultural competency of PSU while improving the research capacity of the community partner to maximize the utility of resources directed towards low-income Latino populations.
3. Identify priority action steps to promote food security and health among low-income producers and consumers of color.

CBPR APPROACH

Increasingly, researchers are using community-based participatory research (CBPR) to address the complex issues associated with racial/ethnic inequities in health (Israel et al. 1998, 2013). CBPR is a collaborative approach to research that facilitates equitable partnership in all phases of the research—from defining the problem to dissemination of findings—and emphasizes power and resource sharing between community and academic partners.

CBPR was a particularly useful approach for the current project because the project involved partners with unique and complementary strengths and resources. Portland State faculty and staff contributed expertise in research methods including survey, focus groups, interviews, and Geographic Information Systems, Adelente Mujeres contributed essential insights into the opportunities and challenges of connecting farmers from its Sustainable Agriculture program with consumers through the local farmers market, and Ecotrust contributed market expertise and connections with institutional buyers in the region. CBPR also facilitated co-learning and capacity building among the partners. Survey development, for example, was an iterative process that fostered a reciprocal exchange of knowledge between the partners; survey questions were initially developed by Portland State University and refined through interaction with Adelente Mujeres staff who were knowledgeable about previous attempts to gather similar information from community members. And by participating in the research process, Adelente Mujeres staff learned how to develop and implement a survey, analyze the data, and disseminate the findings. The project included the use of focus groups, surveys, and Public Participation GIS, which are described below.

Focus Groups

As the initial step of CBPR, Spanish-speaking facilitators from PSU held three focus group sessions to assess community need and capacity. Two of these sessions were with current participating farmers and the last session was with individuals who completed the Adelante Agricultura trainings and had become independent farmers. These sessions uncovered two major themes:

1. The farmers lacked knowledge regarding the produce shopping patterns of local consumers. They wanted more information about what produce to grow and how to market produce as high quality in order to receive a fair price.
2. There was uncertainty among the farmers about local utilization of the Forest Grove Farmers Market. If Forest Grove and Cornelius residents were not utilizing this farmers market, the farmers sought to understand the barriers that were preventing this utilization.

   Other important findings included the challenge of making investments in leased land, the lack of organic certification for the land, the desire to extend the growing season through the use of greenhouses, and the barriers of time (this is typically a secondary economic activity for farmers who work other wage jobs in the area), transportation, and language.

The groups identified several possible solutions: find new sales outlets through connection to institutional buyers and restaurants; get assistance from community partners to connect with other area farmers markets; invest as a group in heated greenhouses or unheated hoop houses; and finally, form a cooperative to share investments and labor and to spread risk.

Market Survey

The focus group findings made it clear that farmers needed more information about local shopping patterns, specifically what products to grow and in what quantities. Farmers were particularly eager for this information because many of the shoppers were non-Hispanic whites, and farmers were not clear on their food preferences. Farmers also wanted to know what shoppers' overall buying patterns were—what would they buy at the supermarket vs. what would they buy at the farmers market? And, could local grocery stores be potential business partners?

PSU students then worked with Adelante staff and clients to develop a quantitative mail survey to collect information from Forest Grove residents about shopping patterns and preferences, as well as residents' familiarity with the Forest Grove Farmers Market. The survey was mailed out to a random sample of 4,000 residents of Cornelius and Forest Grove and received 1,169 responses. PSU students assisted the community partner with analyzing the data using descriptive statistics. Generally, the residents within these communities knew about the Forest Grove Farmers Market. Respondents pointed to a mix of barriers, which created inconveniences for local residents to attend the market (i.e. lack of parking, inconvenient market time, etc.).

Public Participation GIS

The PSU team proposed the use of a Public Participation GIS (PPGIS) approach as a supportive tool to better display the survey findings to Adelante Mujeres staff and community members. The use of PPGIS became a key research contribution and will therefore be discussed at some length here. Despite its status as an emerging field, PPGIS has already demonstrated its potential to serve public health goals. Used by public health practitioners as a community engagement tool, community members have employed PPGIS in identifying determinants of health. This engagement tool has also allowed epidemiologists and policy makers to visualize health disparities that have been identified by a community (Steinberg et al. ND). This visualization creates the ability for these stakeholders to quickly recognize spatial health patterns and can be more successful in conveying messages to the general public than exhaustive statistics and tables.

Because it creates visual information, GIS can enhance the understanding of complex issues and ultimately spur a greater degree of community participation (Salter et al. 2009). However, as the field of GIS has matured, it has tended to meet the needs of an already established technician audience rather than serve as an accessible tool for community members (Talen 2000). Still, many scholars and practitioners recognize that GIS has the potential to be a tool that enhances citizen involvement in public policy and planning issues (Schlossberg and Shuford 2005). Public Participation Geographic Information Systems (PPGIS) thus seek to combine technology-based spatial analysis with grassroots community engagement (Talen 2000; Schlossberg and Shuford 2005). As open source spatial platforms such as Google Earth continue to improve and become more accessible to the general public, an increasing number of public participation efforts are attempting to include Geographic Information Systems (GIS) components. PPGIS has now entered into a variety of fields such as community planning, public health, and education. Unfortunately, of the array of published PPGIS projects, relatively few have focused on community health (Hassan 2005; London et al. 2011; Minkler 2010).

The PSU team knew that PPGIS could work well in this project and would help improve the value of the survey results for identifying ways to improve market outreach efforts. Each survey response was geocoded in order to map responses and look for patterns based on such variables as proximity to the market.

Geographic mapping was possible because each returned survey was connected with the address of that survey participant. A GIS team consisting of three Masters in Urban and Regional Planning graduate students was introduced to complete the mapping portion of the project. The team hoped that analyzing each response according to a specific location could provide spatial patterns that were overlooked by the initial analysis. In addition, the PSU team believed that presenting the data in such a visual form could spark new ideas and conversations regarding the themes that have been brought up within the ongoing CPBR process.

After the creation of the initial categorized points maps, there were significant spatial relationships found between two variables: (1) Those who have heard of the Forest Grove Farmers Market versus those who have not, (2) those who have heard of the Forest Grove Farmers Market and have attended at least once versus those who have heard of the Forest Grove Farmers Market and have never attended. The team created categorized points maps to highlight awareness and utilization of the Forest Grove Farmers Market. The point's maps were layered on top of a zoning map.

To highlight the spatial relationship between these two variables, the GIS team created choropleth maps[2] from the second database that held survey response counts by census tract (normalized by total survey counts in each census tract). There was an obvious west to east spatial relationship between these variables. Our survey data had already indicated that those communities located on the west side of our study area were more likely have heard of and attended the Forest Grove Farmers market. This west to east pattern was not entirely surprising because the Forest Grove Farmers Market was located on the west side of the study area. Nevertheless, the GIS team decided to map demographic census data of our study area to see if this pattern was similar to race or ethnicity disbursement within these cities. By doing so, the team saw a similar west to east pattern with residential patterns by ethnicity, with the Hispanic population concentrated to the east and further from the farmers market.

Further analysis showed the percentage and relative percentage within each census tract of people who listed their ethnicity as Hispanic on the 2010 Census. The west to east pattern is strikingly similar. After deeper analysis of the eastern census tracts, the GIS team found two tracts that stood out. Compared to the other study census tracts, these two had much higher percentages of those who have not heard of the Forest Grove Farmers Market and those who have heard of the Forest Grove Farmers Market and have never attended. These tracts were further away from the market, had less access to public transportation to the area where the market is, and also had higher percentage of Hispanic residents than other tracts in the sample.

ASSESSMENT OF GIS DATA WITH ADELANTE MUJERES

After the survey data were spatially analyzed using ESRI's ArcMap, the results were presented to several Adelante Mujeres representatives. The maps provided a new view of the data that promoted community understanding and discussion. After visualizing the data, Adelante Mujeres staff and clients realized that their uncertainty regarding the underutilization of the Forest Grove Farmers Market was not off base. Additionally, the possible correlation between location of Hispanic residents and the lack of awareness/lack of attendance could have several causes:

1. The outreach efforts (banners, flyers, mail inserts) to increase low-income Hispanic population attendance at the Forest Grove Farmers Market have not been as successful as anticipated.

2. The focus of future outreach/awareness campaigns must target census blocks located on the eastern side of our study area.

The spatial analysis also helped Adelante Mujeres representatives identify potential opportunities and challenges. When analyzing the zoning map, the community members recognized that tract 16 is predominately zoned for single-family residential households. However, tract 13 is zoned for both single-family residential households and multi-family residential households. When it comes to developing future awareness campaigns, these differences become vital. The engagement tactics such as community meetings or canvassing are different when working with multi-family housing units compared to single-family housing units.

Additionally, distance to Forest Grove Farmers Market was discussed. As the maps indicate, those communities that live further than one mile away from the farmers market were less likely to be aware of it or attend. After this pattern was identified, the community partners discussed the possibility of public transit as being a major barrier to access. To eliminate such a barrier, the group discussed the idea of creating a small satellite farmers market near the identified census tracts. Such a development would eliminate the barrier and allow for a stronger presence in the community.

Visualizing these potential opportunities and challenges helped the community partner understand the possible barriers that prevent access to healthy foods which in turn has helped them to be better prepared for future engagement efforts. As can be seen, this spatial data provided a new aspect to the CBPR approach that identified several potential issues that would have been overlooked if this GIS analysis were not brought into the project.

DISCUSSION

The project team helped to improve efforts to increase the participation of low-income Latinos as both producers and consumers of healthy local foods. After verifying that awareness and attendance at the Forest Grove Farmers Market corresponded with both geographic location and ethnicity, PSU students worked with a graphic designer and Adelante Mujeres to develop a logo for the La Esperanza farm. Creating a La Esperanza Farm brand and compelling story helped create awareness of the market and its farmers.

Through the focus group discussions, we identified the farmers' desire to reach new markets and institutional buyers, and were able to connect the farm to other local buyers through Farm to School and Farm to Childcare connections and Ecotrust's Food Hub. Adelante Mujeres developed a relationship with the Farm to School program in the community of study, which holds a high rate of children eligible for free and reduced lunches and large Hispanic population.

The project had other benefits as well. Ecotrust was able to increase their cultural capacity to work with low-income Latino farmers. By facilitating discussions among Latino farmers, the project improved efforts for farmers to work together to solve production and distribution challenges.

Despite progress, the project encountered a number of challenges. Staff turnover among the partners made it difficult to sustain momentum and turn research findings into action plans. For the farmers, the lack of land ownership made it difficult for them to access credit and invest in farm improvements. Time was also a barrier for farmers who also worked other jobs. As low-income earners, we learned that they had a very low tolerance for risk, making it difficult for them to experiment with new crops or market strategies. Limited computer access and the language barrier also made it difficult to take full advantage of the opportunity to use Food Hub to sell their produce.

Ultimately, the study found that the use of PPGIS as a supportive tool was highly successful in complementing an alternative participatory technique; specifically CBPR. Additionally, the application of PPGIS opened up new avenues of discussion and did not create any barriers to participation. The GIS analysis introduced within this study created a new approach to analyzing food environments. Instead of highlighting the location of stores and then identifying the demographic/behavioral patterns of the surrounding communities, this analysis reversed that approach. This study began by understanding the behaviors/demographic patterns of community members based on where they lived. Once behavioral and demographic patterns were understood, then tactics were developed to try to adjust the surrounding food environment (Forest Grove Farmers Market) to these identified patterns. The ability to shape the food environment to the characteristics of the community is a new approach that needs to be explored further.

Additionally, the introduction of the GIS analysis enhanced the CBPR approach. First, the spatial analysis was able to take a limited quantitative survey and identify several patterns by relating responses to residential location. Second, by mapping these identified patterns and displaying them for Adelante Mujeres, new conversations emerged regarding future approaches to increase overall utilization of the Forest Grove Farmers Market in order to boost the consumption of healthy, locally grown produce. Third, the use of GIS helped the research team and community members visualize residential and consumer knowledge patterns in a way that increased participation and furthered dialogue. The introduction of spatial analyses and tools that are typically confined to the occupations of urban planners and geographers shows the increased need for collaborative multidisciplinary research efforts within the realm of public health.

The focus groups, survey data, and GIS analysis all helped the lead organization, Adelante Mujeres, better understand the challenges and limitations of finding markets for their farmers' produce within the local community. A number of important changes have occurred with Adelante Mujeres programming since the end of the CBPR project. First, the organization decided not to renew their lease for La Esperanza farm and ceased operating the farm when the lease expired in 2014. They were able to gain organic certification for the farm, a concern which was raised by farmers during the focus group sessions, but Adelante Mujeres found maintaining certification difficult due to cost and also the challenge of ensuring that all participating farmers maintained careful records required in order to keep the certification. Other factors included the quality of the land, water access issues, and difficulties the organization encountered in managing interpersonal conflicts among the farmers.

With a better understanding of markets, access to institutional buyers through their connections to Ecotrust and others, and their own experience, Adelante Mujeres applied for and received a USDA Community Food Projects program grant in 2013 to establish the Adelante Mujeres Distributor and Community Supported Agriculture (CSA) program. They started the Distributor in 2012 and the CSA in 2013. This allowed the organization to shift approaches. Rather than providing access to land and equipment, Adelante Mujeres provides market access by purchasing produce grown by farmer participants and sells it wholesale to schools, institutional kitchens, restaurants, and higher-end grocery stores, as well as to individuals. This multifarm model provides Latino farmers with market access as well as training opportunities for farmers.

This project confirmed that Latinos often face significant barriers in accessing nutritious, affordable food in their communities, but added important insights about the dynamics of market access for low-income producers as well. By bringing together efforts to improve food access with economic development programs in a low-income Latino community, the project partners sought to reduce obesity and chronic disease and provide avenues for economic development. If the causes of the nutrition transition and the rise in obesity and chronic disease are rooted in a food system that privileges large-scale production and cheap, low-quality foods, reversing the trend will require scalable programs that improve access for low-income consumers and producers alike. A better understanding of how local food markets work and the barriers that low-income producers face in participating in the burgeoning local food systems is an important though often less-visible aspect of improving community nutrition and health.

NOTES

1. The term "Latino/a" and "Hispanic" will be used interchangeably throughout the chapter. Although "Hispanic" is a very general term to represent those populations that descend from a Spanish speaking land or culture, we must use it along with "Latino/a" because federal agencies categorize much of the data for Latino populations under the term "Hispanic."

2. A choropleth map is a thematic map that uses shading to represent average values for geographic areas, such as census tracks or zip codes.

Chapter 9

Religious Gardens, Pilgrimages, and Dancing

A Critique of Translated Interventions in a Tribal Community

Sean Bruna

This chapter addresses theory and practice regarding type 2 diabetes management and prevention at Ysleta del Sur Pueblo (YDSP), a federally recognized American Indian tribe in El Paso, Texas. Type 2 diabetes is a serious and growing concern at the Pueblo, and while the incidence is not as high as in other tribes in the United States, it is still much higher than the national average. Despite excellent biomedical research that shows how individuals can prevent diabetes and countless "translated" diabetes prevention programs that modify evidence-based science for application and use with individuals and families, the incidence of diabetes continues to rise. Drawing from an eight-year partnership and 18 months of community based participatory research with an American Indian Tribe, this chapter critiques current models regarding health intervention, suggests promoting emergent practices from tribal communities rather than continued use of generic "translated" interventions, and provides policy recommendations for application with American Indian and Alaska Native peoples.

In the first section of the chapter I conceptualize "translational" theory and explore what I call "emergent models" of diabetes prevention. In the second section of the chapter I draw on ethnographic research to argue that because religious community gardens, pilgrimages and dancing are practiced by large numbers of the YDSP Tribe's population, and because these activities promote physical activity and healthier eating in a manner that is acceptable to the community, they have the potential to become successful components of wellness programs for obesity and diabetes. I close the chapter with a short discussion regarding policy considerations for integrating the efforts of indigenous leaders and community health staff so that emergent practices can be identified and supported.

ABOUT YSLETA DEL SUR PUEBLO

Ysleta del Sur Pueblo is located in the southeast quadrant of El Paso, TX, along the U.S.-Mexico border. The Pueblo was granted federal recognition in 1987 and shortly thereafter began developing health programs for enrolled members and non-tribal spouses. In 1993, a centrally located building on the reservation was remodeled and repurposed to become the Community Health Center. For the first time, enrolled tribal members had access to a dental clinic, direct-care medical services, and behavioral health programs. In 1996 a modest health education program was added and, with the support of funds from tribal gaming operations, eventually transitioned into the Pueblo's Diabetes Program. Now in its 14th year, the Diabetes Program is combating a slow but steady increase in incidence of the disease across the urban reservation. Of the 1,615 enrolled members, 140 (8.7%) are diagnosed with type 2 diabetes, and for the last several years approximately one new patient has been diagnosed with type 2 diabetes every six weeks. If the incidence of diabetes continues at current estimated rates, it is likely that by 2050 at least one in three individuals on the reservation—including minors—will be diagnosed with type 2 diabetes (Boyle 2010).

REVIEW AND RECONCEPTUALIZATION OF "TRANSLATIONAL THEORY"

There are currently two dominant models, and one emerging model, of diabetes research and intervention among American Indian peoples. Located on a spectrum, they are: (1) individual-oriented biomedical models developed predominately for white, Western populations that are applied both to the general U.S. population and to American Indian peoples; (2) modifications, adaptations, or translations[1] of these programs for application in non-white communities, including American Indian communities; and (3) emerging models of communal prevention in which intervention activities come from local cultural practices and are then enhanced with biomedical practices.

The first model has a historical foundation of individual-oriented clinical research, usually on white populations or what Henrich, Heine, and Norenzayan (2010) have recently recognized in behavioral health research as "Western, educated, industrialized, rich, and democratic cultures," or WEIRD cultures. In most health studies and interventions, the authors argue, minority participants are not represented, so, because so many of the studies and care practices stem from this unrepresentative population, it is likely that researchers either miss important variations and practices or wash over them altogether.

The second dominant model builds on the first by embedding "cultural" modifications, adaptations, or translations of biomedical clinical research for application in non-white communities. These programs are implemented in a more nuanced manner because of the inclusion of various cultural practices, however defined, in the health interventions. However, I argue these programs rely on the ideologies and practices gleaned from research with WEIRD populations and not from the local populations, including indigenous peoples. As I explain, these programs add local indigenous cultural practices into interventions in order to imbue the WEIRD interventions with local practices. The assumption is that by embedding the programs with "culture," the interventions will become more engaging or palatable for the populations they serve. However, in these programs culture becomes an object that stands for, yet masks, the fields where meaningful action and engaging culture practice could take place (Ferzacca 2012). Closer observation of these programs shows that if the programs were implemented in non-tribal settings they would not differ greatly from their tribal counterparts (Joe and Frishkopf 2006).

Individual-Oriented Biomedical Models

Major advances in diabetes prevention occurred in the early 2000s, when the focus of diabetes research shifted to understanding the many different symptoms and individual risk factors of type 2 diabetes in order to design more effective protocols to counter the disease. In a series of landmark studies conducted by the Diabetes Prevention Program Research Group (DPP), clinical researchers found that diabetes could be prevented or delayed. DPP was a randomized clinical trial funded by multiple components of the NIH, with the National Institute of Diabetes and Digestive and Kidney Diseases (NIDDK) as the lead agency (Knowler et al. 2002). From 1996 to 2001, this groundbreaking study sought to determine whether lifestyle intervention or pharmacological therapy with metformin[2] would prevent or delay the onset of diabetes in individuals with impaired glucose tolerance (IGT) who are at high risk for the disease (Ferzacca 2012). The published results indicated that individual-oriented lifestyle intervention reduced the incidence of diabetes by 58% and metformin use reduced the incidence by 31%, as compared with a placebo.

Largely because of the success of biomedical clinical studies that explored the symptoms, risk factors, and methods for preventing or delaying diabetes, programs focused increasingly on individual care and management. The National Diabetes Education Program (NDEP), founded in 1997 to "improve diabetes management and outcomes, [and] promote early diagnoses," paved the way for the institutionalization of individual-oriented biomedical practices in the United States (2011). Based largely on these landmark studies, the National Diabetes Education Program (NDEP) focused in part on increasing individual awareness of A1C, blood pressure, and cholesterol targets—what it called the "ABCs of diabetes." By targeting middle-aged and older Americans, the NDEP hoped to (a) increase awareness of risk factors for type 2 diabetes and diabetes risk tests; (b) increase awareness that type 2 diabetes can be prevented by taking small steps to reduce body weight; and (c) increase knowledge of the four fundamental ways to control diabetes: holding to a diet with less fat and carbohydrates and more vegetables and fruits, increasing regular physical activity, taking medications as prescribed, and working with the health care team to address standard issues as well as complications (NDEP 2013; Clark et al. 2001).

The individual-oriented biomedical model of diabetes management and prevention focused on clinical research and resulted in individual-oriented biomedical practices. These programs are important because they provide essential skills for individuals to prevent or manage diabetes. However, incidence of the disease continues to rise, particularly among American Indian populations. Largely for this reason, research regarding diabetes in American Indian communities has expanded to include a second model that aims to enhance interventions by embedding them with relevant cultural practices.

To address the growing incidence of diabetes in American Indian communities a model with a variety of what may be called "culturally embedded" interventions became more prominent. This model examines the beliefs and practices of local native peoples regarding health and wellness, and the etiology of diabetes, to enhance interventions. These programs, discussed below, attempt to blend biomedical models of health and wellness for prevention and management of diabetes with local indigenous ideologies and "culture." Within these studies, I argue, "culture" is often portrayed in static terms and is believed to be divisible into discrete and static elements such as a clan emblem, a talking circle, or other distilled values, beliefs, or tradition (Engbretson, Mahoney, and Carlson 2008). Although some studies problematize these static portrayals (Ferrira and Lang 2006), the cultural elements are frequently viewed as constant, persistent, and "reversible social and lifestyle factors" (Lancet 2010, 2193). Regrettably, acceptance of this static use of culture hinders program innovation. The programs I discuss below may be more effective than strictly individual-oriented biomedical approaches, but they have yet to expand beyond individual care practices and in most cases are simply Western practices that embed an abstracted cultural practice into a group setting.

In the 1990s and 2000s, researchers began to recognize that the strictly individual-oriented biomedical model of diabetes care and prevention was not resonating with American Indian ideologies concerning health and wellness. Many of the programs in place in American Indian communities promoted Western medical models in which health is solely the responsibility of the individual (Link and Phelan 1995; Raphael, Curry-Stevens and Bryant 2008). These ideologies often conflict with various American Indian cultural practices or beliefs are which holistic, in which the physical body, mind, spirituality/religion, and environment are interconnected (Hodge et al. 2009; King, Smith, and Gracey 2009). As such, an imbalance in one or all of these factors can be understood as the cause of ill health, and a change in one component may impact another.

Despite advances in understanding the local context of diabetes, most programs in the 2000s continued to develop protocols that focused on individual-oriented models, only they were embedded with what were perceived as local cultural practices. Consider the following examples, which embedded the underpinning individual-oriented biomedical model with thinly understood local cultural practices.

The Lionel R. John Health Center/The Seneca Health Trail Blazers/Trails of the Iroquois embedded cultural practices into their programs in an attempt to make them relate to their patient population, but did so in a limited manner. Clinicians asked participants to attend weekly social support sessions and track their educational progress with the assistance of a "clan animal" (Edwards and Patchell 2009). Using a large board, participants moved an image of the animal across a map of the state of New York along a trail from the tribal territory to those of other tribes across the state. As participants progressed through the classes they were also given leather and beading supplies to make mementos to remind them of their weight loss goals and other desired outcomes. Although the program did make strides to understand an important cultural practice—clan animals—it used them in a manner that verged on inappropriate (because clan affiliations are more significant than simple images might imply).

The Sandy Lake School-based diabetes prevention program was a curriculum-based intervention for Ojibwe-Cree students in the third, fourth, and fifth grades (Saksvig et al. 2005) that also touted being "culturally appropriate." Adaptions included the incorporation of local themes such as feasts, "learning from elders," and the use of storytelling as a way to introduce the main concepts of the health education lessons. The stories introduced the diabetes curriculum by following the activities of "Missy and Buddy Daaybway" as they learned from an older family relative about the importance of living a healthy lifestyle to prevent diabetes (Saksvig et al. 2005). To test the effectiveness of the intervention, the study utilized a pre- and post-test, single-sample design conducted during the 1998–1999 school year. The results showed significant increases in dietary intention and preference, knowledge, and dietary self-efficacy. This program showed an improved knowledge related to healthy eating and dietary fiber intake of students in this remote First Nations community, and while it incorporated an enhanced link to local cultural understandings, it is still based on a modification of other interventions.

Finally, a Ho-Chunk Youth Fitness Project in Wisconsin (Carrel et al. 2005) aimed at dietary and exercise instruction and intervention involved 38 Ho-Chunk children and non-native children between 6–18 years of age. The community-based intervention consisted of twice-weekly classes with supervision for both nutrition and exercise. All of the children went through preliminary and post-24-week evaluations that consisted of a medical exam, a nutrition and exercise assessment, metabolic testing of fasting plasma insulin, and measurement of plasma glucose, plasma cholesterol, and percent body fat. Mean fasting plasma insulin levels decreased for the intervention population, and the researchers concluded that supervised nutrition and exercise classes were an effective means to reduce the risk of insulin resistance and the onset of type 2 diabetes.

Each of the programs presented showed an enhanced understanding of local cultural practices that were integrated into a diabetes prevention curriculum. And while they were more nuanced than the individual-oriented biomedical models, they are based, at their foundation, on Western ideologies of health and wellness. Each focused on individual prevention and drew upon practices that were not from the community. They are based, at their foundation, on Western ideologies of health and wellness. In contrast to these two models, a new model of care is developing: emergent communal prevention practices.

"Emergent" Prevention Practices

In contrast to the two models for diabetes care presented earlier, interventions have pushed beyond individual-oriented biomedical models or culturally embedded models to explore an emergent model in which communal emic wellness practices are harnessed for local programs (Baldridge 2001; Satterfield, Burns and Baldridge 2008; Brownstein 2007; Wilson and Satterfield 2007). Among many native peoples, knowledge is intimately linked to local cultural practices. Public health researchers have recognized these knowledge systems and have developed programs which facilitate sharing of success stories concerning healthy foods, tribal histories (Conti 2006; Dapice 2006), and opportunities for changes in diet (Satterfield and Reid 2003). In addition, such emergent interventions have explored metaphor and storytelling to examine the culturally specific meanings that underlie diabetes and diabetes management (Hagey 1984).

In this emerging model, interventions are shifting from individual oriented and broadly focused community-wide interventions to programs that focus on subpopulations within Indian communities, enabling researchers to consider local cultural practices in greater detail. Focusing on subgroups, such as mothers, provides theoretical space for recognizing that cultural practices are never static, a concern which has been voiced by several researchers (Satterfield et al. 2007). In one study with American Indian elders, for example, the author identified two divergent models of diabetes in terms of health behaviors and cultural identification (Henderson 2010). One model was characterized by delayed care-seeking and a negative evaluation of adherence to diabetes self-care. Elders perceived lack of adherence to medical recommendations as a socially acceptable action because adherence placed the elder outside his or her peer group. Early care-seeking and improved adherence to diabetes self-care characterized the second model. These divergent models of diabetes, in which care-seeking, diabetes self-care, and adherence vary as a function of immersion within cultural practices, have implications for health education and disease management and may contribute substantially to health disparities.

In recent years, the agricultural practices of Southwestern Native peoples have been explored independent of health research, often within the framework of tribal sovereignty (Nabhan 2002; Vlasich 2005), and a number of wellness programs are using this agricultural research as part of health interventions. Several diabetes programs are examining the use of gardens as sites for diabetes education. Gardens and farm fields have been essential components in American Indian life for thousands of years. Recently these small-scale agricultural locations have been defined as "community gardens."[3]

Gardens are appealing to the people who design interventions because they engage with local cultural practices and histories while meeting the goals of diabetes prevention programs. In a pivotal commentary on how food choices have become colonized, Devon Mihesuah (2003) proposed using changes in diets and community gardens as a way to decolonize or de-Westernize food options in American Indian communities. In an eloquent section titled "Why Return to Our Gardens?" the author proposes numerous ways to make eating habits healthier, including "Planting and cultivating gardens large enough to feed our families and to keep us active." Though some of the suggestions are unrealistic for families with working parents, the research served as an opening for a discussion connecting diabetes prevention, management, and gardening or farming.

The White Earth Land Recovery Project (WELRP) at the White Earth Reservation of Ojibwe in northern Minnesota (Omura 2006) was an innovative program that addressed type 2 diabetes prevention utilizing gardens. The program sought to build a locally grown food program to assist individuals with diabetes, particularly elders. From the community's perspective, diabetes is a symptom of colonization and is best addressed through decolonizing holistic approaches to food production and related support activities, including development of cookbooks and engagement at powwows. These Ojibwe tribal practices are part of a resurgence of tribal identity on the reservation. As explained by one individual affiliated with the program, "It's not just a medical program, and it's not just a preventative health program . . . it's a cultural restoration program." Rather than adapt a program by embedding it with isolated or decontextualized aspects of the local culture, this program begins with local cultural practices and expands to meet the biomedical needs of diabetes prevention and wellness through decolonizing practices that impact the entire community.

The programs developed as part of the emergent model of diabetes care and prevention is different from the earlier models in many regards. First, they build on activities that are already present in the communities, whether traditional agricultural practices or contemporary youth activities. Second, each of these programs recognizes that cultural practices, like the individuals that shape it, are not static, and as such a variety of practices should be provided for diabetes management and prevention. Third, the programs are unique because a wide variety of community members from across the reservations are engaged in the activities. For example, in the Earth Land Recovery Project, some individuals are involved with farming and harvest activities, others with distribution, while others are consumers.

The emerging model for care and prevention, communal prevention practices, has the potential to engage communities in a manner that is more accepting and more successful than that found in previous research. Although gardens are the first concrete practice to emerge, there are undoubtedly countless other possibilities. This chapter explores this potential by examining the individual-oriented biomedical models and emerging models at play at YDSP.

EMERGENT PRACTICES AT YSLETA DEL SUR PUEBLO

Based on my own ethnographic research, I argue that because religious community gardening, pilgrimages and dancing are practiced by large numbers of the YDSP's population, and because these activities promote physical activity and healthier eating in a manner that is acceptable to the community, they have the potential to become successful components of wellness programs for obesity and diabetes. In contrast to purely individual-oriented biomedical practices, examination of the broader Pueblo community reveals that Pueblo members do participate in many community-wide activities that may prove useful for diabetes prevention. Although the tribal community does not view these activities as wellness practices, if these activities were supported by the Health Center in a culturally appropriate manner that is sensitive to secrecy regarding religious knowledge and other local norms, they could potentially act as effective diabetes prevention practices. These activities emerge from religious institutions and include community gardens and tribally grown food to support nutritional education, religious dancing and pilgrimage activities which promote regular exercise, and enhancement of the Pueblo's built environment to make engagement in wellness activities easier.

Casino Era Wellness Pursuits

During the Pueblo's era of federal recognition (1960–1992), tribal leadership focused its attention on infrastructure and economic development. Individuals moved from the old "Barrio de los Tiguas" to a newly formed reservation with housing built with Housing and Urban Development (HUD) funds. In 1993, following a boom in gaming revenue, the leadership was able to expand housing opportunities for the tribal members and hoped to improve wellness opportunities as well with the construction of tennis courts, an Olympic-sized pool, and a Wellness Center that contained a weight room and multi-purpose dance rooms. Tribal leadership anticipated that these community facilities would be used regularly, ultimately contributing to the health and wellness of the population. Though state of the art, these facilities were underutilized and were slowly scaled down beginning in 2009. In 2012 the pool closed and the space was converted into an entertainment center. The programs and services that were developed during the casino era were never utilized anywhere near capacity. The pool and wellness facilities were designed by an outside consulting firm to enhance the exercise opportunities for Pueblo residents, but they never considered that local approaches to wellness were different than that of the surrounding non-native populations. This may be why the facilities failed to attract members and ultimately closed. Ironically, the cost to maintain the pool, an estimated $40,000 per month, is slightly less than the estimated cost of care for four diabetic patients (Javitt and Chiang 2013).

In contrast, there are community wellness practices that *are* culturally accepted and *communal*. These include gardens, religious pilgrimages, and religious dancing. I call these activities *communal* rather than *community* activities because they are practiced and experienced simultaneously by groups of individuals rather than individually.

Religious Pilgrimages

Each year in early June, community members gather at a small, inconspicuous residential lot about a quarter mile from the Pueblo's mission to hold the Salida de los Santos (Presentation of the Saints) pilgrimages. If promoted appropriately by the Pueblo, this activity could align with the goals of diabetes prevention program because it is an excellent form of exercise.

A pilgrimage is "a journey to a special place, in which both the journey and the destination have spiritual significance for the journeyer" (Davidson and Gitlitz 2002). The Salida de los Santos pilgrimage, as explained by Montaña, the Pueblo's religious leader, is a tradition dating back to the time when the area was primarily a farming community. On this day, the images of Saint Anthony de Padua are carried in the four directions by members of the Tribe for the blessing of the farm fields and houses in the area. Today, the same traditional routes are followed as the Santos is carried from house to house. Persons wishing to welcome the Santos into their homes may do so and receive a house blessing. In addition, offerings of money or food (canned or dry) are made to the Santos. The *limosna* (money offerings) are used to pay for the mass, choir, flowers, church decorations, and *vestiture* (ceremonial dress) of the San Antonio idol for the feast day on June 13. They are also used to purchase food for the public community meal served that day. Food donated is given to needy families in the area.

At this unassuming yet deeply significant place, two canals intersect and stretch out in the four cardinal directions. Montaña explained that this was where the members of the Pueblo stayed when they arrived in the El Paso region following the Pueblo Revolt. Each year the residents of the Pueblo meet at this location to honor that night. They divide into four groups, either to walk with families or to pick a route that they enjoy or are able to walk, and process along the canals in the four directions. Pilgrimages such as Salida, as Yvette, a coordinator with tribal youth programs, explained, are one of the most well-attended religious events at the Pueblo, and one of the few events in which community members participate as families, not individuals. Another individual walking the pilgrimage explained that different families lead the different walks and pass this responsibility to relatives each year.

The four routes extend into different neighborhoods, roughly in the four cardinal directions, and are known for the community they traverse as well as their varying difficulty. The southern route is called El Garrote (the club), and the walks take place along the neighborhood located near the Tuh-lah. To the west is Ysleta 1, a densely packed residential area, and to the east is Ysleta 2. The route to the north is called San Jose, and it passes the San Jose Church toward the northernmost boundary of the Pueblo's original land grant. This is the route that I traveled two years in a row, and which I discuss below.

Preparations for Salida began on June 3, the day before the pilgrimages. Women gathered in the Tuh-Lah and clean six-foot tables and chairs thoroughly with washcloths and solutions of diluted bleach. In the kitchen, meanwhile, food was prepared for the participants of the pilgrimages, including breakfast burritos, brisket, assorted fruit, and an assortment of drinks such as water and Gatorade. On outdoor grills, fat cut from the brisket was grilled or fried for snacks to be eaten while the cooks were working.

Several individuals mentioned that, in 2009, temperatures were in the high 90s, and in 2010 they were expected to be well above 102°F. They encouraged me to drink plenty of water the day before and to eat a light meal. Two men explained that one year they had gone out drinking the night before the event and regretted it. "Man, last year I was drinking the night before and I had a terrible hangover, and it was the most difficult day that I'd had." I learned from others that this was not only a health warning but also lesson about the strict taboo against drinking at all religious events. Other individuals provided more tangible suggestions, urging me to dress in loose-fitting athletic wear[4] and to cancel any interviews or activities the day after the pilgrimage because I would be sore from walking.

On June 4, the day of the Salida, individuals arrived at Nakitu Street, the location of the Tuh-Lah, at 4:00am to prepare breakfast,[5] and individuals wanting breakfast arrived between 4:30 and 6:00am. At 6:00am, all individuals in attendance walked to the church for a short mass. Once we were at the church, Father Charles entered, wearing his formal white regalia. Behind him entered the bishop. Each gave a prayer, and Father Charles smudged all in attendance with a special Pueblo-style smudge pot and an eagle fan.

After approximately half an hour, everyone made their way down the road to Old El Paso and Whitely Street,[6] the site of two intersecting canals, with the traffic redirected by the Tribal Police. Montaña, the war captain, explained that I could take photos once we left the sacred site, but not while we made our way there, or at the site itself. Once there, Montaña gave a prayer and we divided into our four pilgrimage groups. I joined the San Jose group and followed three individuals who led us at a fast walking pace. Yvette carried a small statue of San Antonio and powered on ahead. An individual with a burlap bag flanked her on the right, and on her left an individual continuously rang a brass bell.

As we made our way along the canal and roads, we stopped at houses to invite both tribal and non-tribal members to the Feast Day, offered a blessing for their home, and collected donations of beans, canned goods, or cash. Between the clangs of the brass bell, Montaña told me "that this walk was actually done to bless the fields and the houses; that even up to 20–30 years ago the area was nothing but fields, so it was to bless the fields for good harvests and growth, to bless the houses."

As we weaved through the streets and canals, we came upon different plants, and Montaña occasionally pulled me aside to show me their use. "These are *garambullos,*" he explained. "Wolf-berries, I think." He handed me some quarter inch, round, grape-looking fruits that were growing on vines along the ditches. Soon, others circled around to hear what was being said and began to pick them off the vine. "We used to make jelly out of these and spread them on bread," Montaña explained before we continued on our way.

By 11:00am, it was already 92°F and the temperature was steadily rising. We continued walking, and at certain points, instructed by individuals with walkie-talkies, trucks would arrive with the tribal grounds staff to hand out water and Gatorade, and to shuttle individuals back and forth to use the restroom. For lunch we stopped to rest under two weeping willow trees that were planted by the tribe several years ago. Tribal support staff arrived again and individuals handed out lunch, consisting of beef brisket burritos, an extra flour tortilla, a bag of Sun Chips, a granola bar, and a small baggie with either grapes or cherry tomatoes. Coke, Gatorade, or water was offered, and most individuals chose to drink both soda and water. Vegetarians were offered hash brown burritos instead of brisket.

After lunch we continued on what became a gruelingly difficult pilgrimage. The temperature peaked at 107°F, a record-setting day for the year. We continued on, and at one point I was passed the bell and asked to join the group. "Come on Mr. Sean, we have to pick the pace up!" Yvette encouraged as I walked alongside her, the bell slowly feeling heavier and heavier. Eventually, we reached what I am told was the midpoint of our route, a small agricultural hill where a farmer planted corn and red chile. Hidden behind a Wal-Mart and a convent, the field seemed out of place, isolated from the bustle of El Paso. A handful of individuals walked to the top of the hill and stopped at the last house on the route. They returned several minutes later, and the rest of the group slowly began to make their way back.

We returned to the Tuh-Lah a little after 3:00pm and were greeted by lines of applauding CHRs and cooks. "Thank you for your sacrifice!" Diego said to several individuals before shuttling them to tables for a meal of freshly baked bread, peas with red chile, spaghetti, beans with *chicharrones* (pork rinds), tea, and water. A new drink option, pineapple juice, watermelon juice, or lemonade, rounded out the selection and was handed out by the CHRs. In time, the three other groups arrived and also enjoyed freshly cooked meals.

This pilgrimage is deeply significant to YDSP because of the connection to the place and because it initiates the activities for the religious feast. However, in addition to its religious significance, this activity provides a valuable educational lesson for diabetes prevention and wellness. The event promotes physical activity and welcomes all individuals from the Pueblo to participate. In addition, the food that is offered at the event is culturally appropriate and portioned into healthy servings, while water is offered alongside other sugar based beverages.

Religious Dancing

Pueblo dancing is one of the most important activities at a Pueblo, and it is deeply significant for the individuals who dance, those who help prepare for the event behind the scenes, and those who are spectators. Religious dancing is a process that unfolds over time and connects dancers with each other, their Pueblo origins, and spiritual realms in what may be called a ritual drama, or a "process which serves to unite humans with other humans, as well as humans with other-than-humans, the revealed with the unrevealed worlds, the visible with the invisible" (Frisbie 1980).

Eleven religious dances take place at the Pueblo on nearly a monthly basis. The religious dance calendar is shaped by agricultural practices and is so significant that it regulates political terms for the Tribal Council. Based on syncretism of Catholic and Native religious practices stemming back to 1680s, dances are named after Catholic saints and involve a mix of Catholic rituals at the church in addition to the dancing. It is unethical to discuss specific dance practices, such as dance steps and *figuras* (formations), in deference to privacy restrictions enforced by the tribe to protect their cultural knowledge. However, some general practices may be described and are useful for understanding the intersection of dance and wellness.

Dances at YDSP begin with tribal members meeting at the Tuh-lah at or before dawn. Upwards of 80 dancers currently participate in the Feast Day dance (with 50 or more individuals providing support), whereas smaller dances may have only 20 dancers. Since completion of the kiva in 2009, members meet inside the kiva for prayer and, in some cases, dance before moving to the main dance ground. In general, a spectator to a public dance at the Pueblo would see a rectangular area with a group of male "chanters" (singers) circled behind the Pueblo's red sacred hand-held drum, a sun painted on one side and a moon on the other. To the left and right of the men are two shoulder-to-shoulder rows of dancers, men on one side, and women on the other. At the four corners around the dancers stand four *capitanes* (captains) with pump-action shotguns. These individuals serve two purposes. While dances are taking place, they form a spiritual boundary around the dancers, and while dancers are in transit on city streets between one dance ground and another, they assist with traffic control, firing at or above cars if they do not stop.

Approximately 15 chanters (more, if available) sing while two or three individuals hold the tribe's sacred drum with a rope suspension while another individual beats the drum and leads the song. Songs are sung or chanted in a mix of Tiwa and Spanish and provide a rhythmic downbeat for the dancers. At given points in the song, the pairs of men and women come together and dance in a manner that represents planting. Men move as if opening the soil with a planting stick, and women follow with a motion of throwing seeds on the soil and covering the hole with a quick shuffle of their feet. Dancers complete sets of dances until everyone has completed dancing or a specific dance pattern has been completed. At YDSP, some dances move back and forth between the traditional dance ground and a plaza in front of the Catholic church, and at designated moments the dancers form specific *figuras*.[7] At lunchtime (usually around noon) dancers take a break and enter the Tuh-lah's cafeteria for a communal meal. Dancers continue until dusk, at which point they complete their dances and ceremonies.

Individuals dance for many reasons and see it as a way to pray for others. Many individuals make a *promesa* (promise) in which they vow to dance and pray for another individual. When they dance, they "dance hard," which can be described as being committed to the dance and committed to others in a positive and loving manner.

All of the dances are deeply significant and have specific meanings, though it is inappropriate to discuss the meaning and significance in detail. In general terms, dancers always recognize the four cardinal directions, the air above them, and land below them, and a ceremonial center that where all elements and directions meet. The four directions represent the four seasons, tying the Pueblo in both time and space, and individuals honor the four directions when they dance, thus tying themselves to each other, the Pueblo, and the broader landscape.

Individuals participate in feasts as a way to pray, to honor their Pueblo identity, and to recognize membership at YDSP. By participating in the dance or assisting in the kitchen, individuals learn about cultural patrimony, language, and other specific practices that are not actively documented or learned in written form. Participants support each other, rather than standing out as individuals, and in doing so create a profound experience that is shared by all involved.

Dancing requires an incredible amount of physical endurance. The smaller dances may last between 3 hours and 6 hours, but the larger ones can last up to 10 or 12 hours, as is the case with the St. Anthony Feast Day. To prepare, the best dancers run regularly throughout the year and practice dance steps on their own or with close friends; some minors practice by dancing weekly at the public dances at the cultural center. Prior to dances, community members gather for intensive practice sessions. Prior to the Fiesta de San Antonio, dancers gather for four one- to three-hour practice sessions.

Like the pilgrimage discussed earlier, religious dancing could serve as an effective means to promote the physical activity goals of the Diabetes

Program, but only if it is linked in a culturally appropriate manner that recognizes the deep significance of religious dancing to Pueblo identity, spirituality, and community wellbeing. For example, to prepare for the pilgrimages, the Pueblo could organize weekly walking groups, while more active individuals could join a running club to train for the demanding physical activity required at religious dances. Care should be taken, however, not to overstep or underestimate the religious foundation of the activities by implying that dancing is an activity designed to stay in shape, and not for religious and spiritual purposes.

Religious Gardens and Communal Food

Community gardens have been utilized by other American Indian diabetes prevention programs (Armstrong 2000). These gardening programs are being used to complement or extend biomedical models for diabetes prevention, whereby individuals engage in gardening and learn about individual exercise and nutrition practices. At YDSP, several gardens were developed, but surprisingly, not to serve as central sites for diabetes education or to provide food for nutritional interventions, a common practice in gardens in non-native communities. As time progressed I learned that the significance of the Pueblo gardens was far deeper than I initially expected: unlike gardens that focus exclusively on production of healthy produce for nutritional education programs or to support biomedical education models (Lombard 2006; Mihesuah 2003), the gardens at YDSP were linked to a collection of integrated and deeply significant religious practices that may connect to diabetes prevention in a manner that has been missing from the medical programs utilized by other diabetes prevention programs, including the one at the YDSP. As a member of the Tribal Council said, "A lot of tribal members might not know that dancing is part of the [the agricultural calendar]. To involve and incorporate that information into a diabetes program and the whole community garden is just awesome."

The significance of gardens, their timelines, and how they link to wellness was explained by Montaña. Planting the garden, he explained, took place on Good Friday, or sometime after Easter Sunday, "maybe that's called Easter Monday", he stated. Corn would also be planted, preferably the tribe's white corn that is used at every ceremony. The corn, he said, should be planted the first week of March.

Montaña explained that dances and prayers were held during the first week of March when the irrigation canals were opened. "The acequia madre," he said, pointing in the direction of the canal that ran next to tribal council offices, "was opened up to get water from the Rio. We can't do that anymore because of the border fence and other problems." He paused, gathering his thoughts. "But the church made us farm when we came down here. And by the 1800s there were many vineyards all over." He then went into his closet and pulled out a large photo portfolio. He began flipping through photos, stopping at several that showed oxen being used on the farms, and grapes being harvested and crushed into juice for wine. "See, we used ox for this work. And the church wanted the wine. We also have a wine, our drink . . . it's made with the corn and is called *tesguino*." Montaña continued, "We would like to have other plants, like sage too. I bought a sage in Wal-Mart, but it is not doing so good. It does not grow very big, so maybe with your expertise, some soil testing and the sort, you can tell us how to improve the soil. Maybe we can bring manure from the ranch. We can bring in the BS for good use," he joked as we discussed additional details.

Religious pilgrimages, dancing, and gardening could serve as activities that meet the goals of the diabetes prevention program. Unlike the Olympic-sized pool and gym that were built by external contractors during the gaming era, these long-standing and significant activities are practiced and supported by community members in specific places.

Dances take place throughout the year, and individuals participate as dancers, chanters, cooks, or event staff. With an estimated 80 to 100 dancers currently participating year-round, and 100 to 200 individuals providing support in kitchens, cafeterias, or on the dance grounds, there is an opportunity to align the wellness goals of the diabetes program with food preparation and exercise activities that are already in place and accepted by the community.

The location of the dances and gardens is significant. Historically, Pueblo dance grounds were the center of communities, both literally and metaphorically. Houses surrounded the dance grounds and activities were practiced on them as governed by the agricultural calendar. Ysleta de Sur Pueblo, though an urban pueblo, also had this design prior to becoming urbanized. The Tuhlah was, and still is, surrounded by tribally owned homes. However, when the tribe received federal recognition and HUD funding, the center of the Pueblo shifted from the dance grounds of the Barrios de los Tiguas to the Community Health Center. With that, the central focus of wellness shifted from communal activities, such as religious pilgrimages or dancing on the agricultural calendar, to the individual-centered practices in medical appointments. However, the dance ground, what one member of the Pueblo grounds staff calls "the heart of the Pueblo," is still strong, and, if tied with diabetes prevention in a culturally appropriate manner, as identified through ethnographic research and in depth communication with community members and local stakeholders, has the potential to support physical as well as spiritual wellness for generations to come.

POLICY CONSIDERATIONS

Type 2 diabetes is a serious public health concern for American Indians as well as the general U.S. population. As explained earlier, individual-oriented biomedical care/prevention models are necessary for management of type 2 diabetes. And while individual-oriented biomedical approaches are important, I argue here that researchers should also consider community-specific emergent models of prevention. As Ferreria and Lang explain, we need to examine "the diabetes epidemic with a broader semantic domain that extends well beyond the narrowly defined biologic and genetic condition into the realms of social relations, history, and the politics of Indigenous identity" (2006, 16). In doing so, diabetes prevention efforts become culturally specific and, potentially, more effective. Shifting along the research spectrum from individual-oriented biomedical models to culturally-embedded models to emergent models will not be easy as researchers will need to examine local cultural practices and select those that may prove suitable for integration with diabetes prevention programs. Community gardens have been harnessed in this emergent model, and undoubtedly countless other activities are culturally significant in American Indian and Alaska Native tribes and would be useful in this regard. The challenge is to take the time to engage with communities, ethnographically or otherwise, to explore appropriate opportunities.

This chapter connects with broader debates in anthropology regarding health research with native peoples as well as long-standing topics in anthropology. As an anthropological study of type 2 diabetes, this research questioned who, how, and where we discuss diabetes. Rather than focus on biomedical studies that exclusively address medical professionals and patients within a clinical setting, this research moved outside the clinic to include staff who are not usually considered in health studies: grounds staff, tribal leaders, and religious leaders. By including these individuals the research explored new topics and shed light on new and potentially effective means to prevent diabetes.

In addition to incorporating populations that are usually not included in diabetes prevention research, this research utilized a new set of research technologies. Rather than focusing on glucometers, testing strips, and pedometers, this research utilized traditional religious knowledge, shovels, and irrigation pumps. These research technologies may fall out of the skill set of most researchers, but by not shying away from them, I had the opportunity to form partnerships with the individuals who used them and move the research in a potentially more useful direction.

In part because of new research partners and tools, new and novel diabetes prevention programs may develop at YDSP and may serve as a model for other tribes. The next challenge for the tribal health center, as with health centers everywhere, is to change tribal health policies and internal structural practices that may deter program innovation. For example, YDSP could make it easier to attend religious events by making them paid tribal holidays so that more individuals may attend, or integrate departments that are traditionally distinct, such as health and human services, housing, and tribal grounds. Doing so may alleviate the tendency to isolate and "silo" programs (and their funding) across the reservation, a concern as new diabetes education programs shift outside of the clinic and link with religious or economic development programs, each of which has separate budgets. My hope is that with concerted effort, medical discourses and structures can become permeable so they can incorporate community knowledge and practices.

Finally, as health care practices shift from inside the health centers to communities, care must be taken to ensure that health care policies do not overstep their boundaries regarding privacy or in regards to religious practices. For example, health care practices are increasingly moving towards preventative care, especially following enactment of the Patient Protection and Affordable Care Act (2010). As prevention becomes more prominent in community life, it may be beneficial for tribal health centers to approach emergent practices, particularly those that link prevention efforts to religious practices, cautiously and with regular input from tribal and religious leaders. With these considerations in mind, new programs will not only emerge, but flourish.

NOTES

1. "Translation" is the term used by the National Institutes of Health and the Centers for Disease Control and Prevention for programs and methods that have been modified from the clinical setting for application in "real world" community settings.

2. Metformin is an antidiabetic drug that is given to obese or overweight individuals to help them counter diabetes. It has been shown to reduce complications and mortality rates associated with the disease.

3. The term "community garden" is recent, having been introduced in the United States after World War II. Wills (1988) offers a detailed examination of prehistoric farmers of the American Southwest.

4. Unlike many religious events at the Pueblo, participants in Salida wear street clothing. Kathy, a CHR, instructed me to wear a hat and red bandana around my neck (red being the religious color), good walking shoes and running socks, a moisture-wicking t-shirt, jeans, and mid-length UnderArmor underwear to prevent chafing, all suggestions I was very glad to receive.

5. Mayordomos, or sponsors, managing this event were exceptionally friendly and supportive. Rather than having to bike to the Tuh-Lah, I was picked up by Bear at 3:30am and we arrived to find freshly brewed hot coffee and a selection of Mexican

pastries. Though I struggled to find words at that early hour, the individuals around me seemed cheerful and were able to joke without hesitation.

6. Names have been changed to protect confidentiality of the site.

7. In a variety of dance figuras, dancers create various designs such as a four-pointed star which indicates each of the four directions. Historically, this formation has also been called la estrella (Spanish for "star") and Pa'huitla, the Tiwa word for star. Other dance formations have names as well, though for reasons regarding the privacy and sacredness of the dances, I was asked not to document them.

Chapter 10

Considering Surgical Weight Loss

Applied Anthropology and the Invisible Obese Body

Sarah Trainer, Alexandra Brewis, and Amber Wutich

Anthropological engagement with the "problem" posed by obesity has been growing in recent years. Within this larger engagement, biocultural approaches highlight ecological and evolutionary drivers, including structural inequalities, food preferences, and exposure to psychosocial stress, to name only a few (e.g., Brewis 2011; Brewis et al. 2011; Brown and Konner 1987; Kulick and Meneley 2005; McElroy 1990; Pike 2004; Ritenbaugh 1982; Wells 2010).

Much of the more explicitly ethnographic literature has centered on critiquing the ubiquitous medical and popular admonitions of people and populations classified as overweight and obese, but most of the actual research upon which these critiques are based has occurred within mostly "normal weight" populations working to avoid weight gain (e.g., Greenhalgh 2012; McClure 2013; Nichter 2000; Taylor 2006). Focused ethnographic study with those most affected by the everyday realities of extreme obesity—those who are categorized socially and medically as fat/obese, in other words—remains limited to a handful of small, cross-sectional studies primarily conducted by non-anthropologists (e.g., Carryer 1997; Millman 1980; Rogge 2004; Sobal and Maurer 1999; Thomas et al. 2008). As we have noted elsewhere (Trainer et al. 2015), this lack of systematic, focused ethnographic study of the daily experiences of those most affected by the "obesity epidemic," and the moral panic it elicits (Campos 2004; Saguy 2013), underscores what has been termed the "social invisibility" (Casper and Moore 2009) that obesity appears to create. To be more precise, it seems to exacerbate the lack of voice or opinion allowed to individuals whose bodies are viewed socially and medically as unacceptable, focusing only on the problematic physical body itself.

So what do we know ethnographically about what it is like to live with extreme weight in the United States today? Millman's now three-decades-old work (1980) has been important in detailing how the fat body is integral to definitions of self, so that the two cannot easily be disarticulated. A few other studies have, using small samples, explored the ways in which individuals alternatively absorb and resist stigmatizing, marginalizing, and blaming messages targeting their size (Carryer 1997; Rogge 2004; Sobal and Maurer 1999; Thomas et al. 2008). Struggles to lose weight are detailed in these studies, but the "struggles" are almost inevitably unsuccessful from the point of view of the individuals attempting to lose weight. Furthermore, despite fervent public and medical discourse advocating planet-wide weight loss (Campos 2004, Saguy 2013), nuanced and systematic study of those who actually embark on radical, technologically-driven weight loss programs is likewise largely missing. Fat Studies research does prioritize the voices and experiences of fat men and women within a broader agenda of feminist- and queer-driven writing (Atkins 1998; Braziel and LeBasco 2001; Farrell 2011; Gailey 2012; Kulick and Meneley 2005; Orbach 1978; Rothblum and Solovay 2009). The research does not tend to be systematic or ethnographic in focus, however, instead adhering to a clear political agenda—ending fat-based discrimination.

As anthropologists with a long-standing interest in issues involving obesity, obesity stigma, and body image (Brewis 2014, 2011, 1999; Brewis and Gartin 2006; Brewis and Lee 2010; Brewis and McGarvey 2000; Brewis et al. 2011; Brewis et al. 1997; Brewis and Wutich *forthcoming,* 2015; Hruschka et al. 2011; Maupin and Brewis 2014; Trainer 2013; Trainer et al. 2015; Wutich et al. 2014), we are concerned with this identified lack. In this chapter, we set out to systematically identify and delineate these dimensions of current anthropological research into issues involving obesity. We outline this argument using data obtained from two commonly-used anthropological search engines, Anthrosource and Anthroplus, and we then place this data in the context of our most recent ethnographic work with extremely obese bariatric patients. Based on our interviews and participant observation with and among those who are considering bariatric surgery—a set of surgeries that drastically restructure the stomach and gut, a technological intervention that enables extremely obese individuals to lose weight—we explain how an ethnography of an extremely obese clinical "community" can help to reveal new ways to support people already profoundly affected by the powerful, negative social meanings of obesity/fat.

STUDYING THE EXISTING LITERATURE

We began our work with a systematic literature review of the anthropological literature on obesity, focusing on the past 15 years, excluding publications without English translation. We did this using keyword search in

Anthrosource and Anthroplus, the two main search engines specific to the field of anthropology. Anthrosource is the flagship search engine of the American Anthropological Association, which "indexes current issues for eleven of the AAA's most critical peer-reviewed publications" (AAA 2015). Anthroplus is "a compilation of the *Anthropological Index Online* and *Anthropological Literature* databases . . . [with an] extensive index of bibliographic materials covering the fields of anthropology, archaeology, and related interdisciplinary research" (EBSCO 2015). Keywords were "obese," "obesity," and "fat." In Anthrosource, "obesity" yielded 15 publications, "obese" yielded three publications, and "fat" 25 publications. Anthroplus, "obesity" yielded 1,101 publications; "obese" resulted in 107 hits, and "fat" 1,255. We eliminated anything published before 2000, reviews of other work, or comments.

Based on this search, we found that no publications in Anthrosource included the voices and perspectives of people living with extreme obesity. Typical exemplars of the literature included articles focused on obesogenic environments and policy, and the ways in which policy and larger structural forces encourage obesogenic behaviors (e.g., Brewis 2011; Crooks 2003; Everett and Wieland 2012; Fitzgerald 2010; Himmelgreen et al. 2012; Moffatt 2010; Maupin and Brewis 2014; Wiedman 2012); discussions of hunger-obesity paradoxes, in which we not only see undernutrition and over nutrition existing side-by-side in communities but also affecting the same individual at different points in the lifecourse (e.g., Brenton 2013; Brewis 2011; Dahl 2014; Pike 2013); analyses of increasing anti-fat attitudes across all sectors of societies world-wide (e.g., Brewis 2011; Greenhaulgh 2012); use of obesity to discuss structural inequalities and the ways in which poverty, stress, and lack of opportunity create increased risk of weight gain (e.g., Benson 2012; Chollett 2014); and explorations of the discourses and practices of people worried about gaining weight, especially the phenomenon of "fat talk" (e.g., Nichter 2000).

With Anthroplus, the majority of the search returns were extremely biomedical in orientation, reporting anthropometric measures, population-level BMI increases and lifestyle trends, fat patterning, etc. Others adopted evolutionary frameworks for their discussions of the current "obesity epidemic." At-risk populations (at the national level, the community level, even the level of the family) were highlighted in the publications, but the research overwhelmingly did not have an ethnographic focus. Rather, it concentrated on anthropometric- or survey-derived data on behavior and weight perceptions.

Anthroplus-obtained publications that did use ethnographic methods were limited to discussions of increasing anti-fat attitudes across all sectors of societies worldwide (e.g., Brewis and Wutich 2012; Brewis et al. 2011), reports on perceptions of attractiveness and body fat percentages (e.g., Brewis 2012; Brewis and McGarvey 2000; Dressler et al. 2008; Faries and Bartholomew

2012; Gremillion 2005; Kaufer-Horwitz 2006), comparisons of health-related behaviors and attitudes between normal weight and overweight/obese groups (e.g., Brewis 2003; Hauff and Demerath 2012; Hulens et al. 2002; Poveda et al. 2014), explorations of weight gain and "blame" rhetoric (e.g., Greenhaulgh 2012; Greenhalgh and Carney 2014; Herndon 2010; Lund and Miller 2014; Namie 2011; Warin et al. 2011), articles focused on weight loss (e.g., Booker 2000), and more articles focused on obesogenic environments, nutrition knowledge, and policy (e.g., Brewis 2012; Brewis and Gartin 2006; Brewis and McGarvey 2000; Brown et al. 2009; Bugge 2011; Crooks 2003, 2000; Himmelgreen et al. 2004; Hruschka 2012; Hugo and Franzon 2006; Gartin 2012; Johnston 2006; Moffat 2010; Musaiger et al. 2000; Pérez-Escamilla et al. 2001; Seiden et al. 2012; Young 2007). Once again, the voices of the extremely obese were largely absent from the published narratives: researchers talked *about* obese bodies, or simply talked *to* those same obese bodies long enough to gather behavioral data, without providing a space or opportunity for more in-depth exploration of the people behind the bodies and behaviors identified as at-risk.

The only search results that employed ethnographic methods (particularly in-depth interviewing techniques and participant observation) within populations characterized as morbidly obese were conducted by researchers whose listed departmental affiliations and training were not anthropological. Most commonly, such exceptions were psychologists using in-depth interviewing techniques among obese (e.g., Satinsky 2013) and/or post-bariatric populations (e.g., Meana and Ricciardi 2008). These studies were characterized by small sample sizes and cross-sectional, single interviews. Sociologists also employed ethnographic work, including longitudinal participant observation and in-depth interviews, within organizations such as Overeaters Anonymous, Weight Watchers, and the National Association to Advance Fat Acceptance (e.g., Boero 2012, 2010; Martin 2002), while adopting a more Foucauldian perspective to analyze techniques and narratives around the medicalization and pathologization of large bodies.

Anthropological work explicitly aimed at articulating people's lived experiences and personal perspectives on those experiences thus remains elusive in the existing literature.

CONDUCTING CLINICALLY-EMBEDDED ETHNOGRAPHY

One key site of convergence for many important and current issues in the anthropology of the body is the socially stigmatized, economically excluded, "failed" bodies of the 16 million U.S. adults who struggle daily with morbid obesity (also labeled Class-III Obese, based on BMI/body mass index>=40, see WHO 2014a). We argue that within this group, one of the most focused points of convergence amenable to detailed ethnographic study is the "work in progress" bodies of the 160,000 U.S. adults who every year elect to undergo bariatric surgery, a surgery that allows people, via technological interventions, to lose significant amounts of weight (ASMBS 2013; Mechanick et al. 2013).

Our position as researchers is somewhat unique, inasmuch as the *Obesity Solutions Initiative* in which we are administratively located is a joint endeavor between Arizona State University and Mayo Clinic. As Mayo Clinic affiliates, we have a unique opportunity to directly recruit within a highly regarded and large bariatric practice, affording excellent opportunity to examine the life histories, experiences, and perspectives of those electing bariatric surgery—who must be "extremely obese" from a medical perspective to even qualify for surgery.

For the last 12 months, Trainer has been conducting general participant observation throughout the public areas of Mayo Clinic's hospital and outpatient facilities in Phoenix, observing many of the Mayo Clinic's bariatric team bi-monthly meetings, the required Behavioral Change classes for all pre-operative bariatric patients, and monthly bariatric support group meetings. The classes are supervised by a Mayo Clinic RN and a rotating cadre of Mayo Clinic dieticians and each cycle lasts eight weeks; all patients must attend the classes, as well as meet individually with the RNs, dieticians, surgeons, and psychologist. For reasons stemming from issues of patient privacy and confidentiality, we do not observe the individual clinic encounters, but we have access to all group venues. This sets the context for the detailed narrative interviews with patients themselves. Thus far, we have interviews with 25 individuals, seven men and 18 women. Of these, two of the men identify as Asian-American, two of the women as African-American, one man as Latino, and two other women as Latina; everyone else identifies as White. Two of the men and six of the women are >65 years of age and not formally employed and the others are <65 and employed.

A year into the study, our interview sample is still small and our analysis necessarily still qualitative and preliminary. This highlights the difficulties of working with such a vulnerable population, as well as the intricacies involved in navigating an institutional structure and clinical culture focused on patient care, perhaps explaining why clinically-embedded ethnographies are less frequently conducted by anthropologists than community-based ones (Mikecz 2012). We have thus far focused on inductive theme identification phase of text-based analysis of interview transcripts, supplemented with analysis of fieldnote transcripts (Krippendorff 2012; Wutich et al. 2014).

One of the most powerful findings to emerge from our data thus far is the theme of trauma and stress over a lifetime. Study participants came to the

Mayo bariatric program with an accumulation of lifetime health insults (emotional, social, and physical), some overtly weight-related and some seemingly unrelated. These complaints were often physical: participants reported struggling with joint problems, fibromyalgia, cancer, sleep apnea, menopause, hysterectomies, and pain from physical trauma. In opposition to dominant American narratives that assume all the illnesses that affect an obese body are a result of that obesity (Brewis 2011), many participants clearly made the point that a previous physical traumatic event limited their ability to make healthy choices (including regular exercise) and thus, exacerbated or even precipitated extreme weight gain. Mo, for example, felt that she "spread" alarmingly after a hysterectomy. Alison cited a chronic hormonal imbalance and knee problems as key triggers for her stress eating, inability to be physically active, and tendency to retain weight.

Other participants detailed the physical limitations and pain associated with obesity itself and the ways in which these had severely impacted their well-being over the years. As Todd said, "Each year would get a little worse [in terms of his physical mobility and knee pain]. I didn't know that's what I was doing. I didn't feel that. It's just I did less, went out less, was less sociable, was more irritable."

Complaints could also be emotional. Participants discussed long-term emotional trauma related to closed adoptions, familial suicides, abusive romantic relationships, and childhood poverty. Many again made the connection between emotional trauma and a later inability to properly manage their health. At the same time, participants did detail the ways in which being "fat" resulted in discrimination and felt stigma, whether in romantic relationships, relationships with family members or friends, or in the workplace. This complicated, multi-directional flow between trauma and obesity and trauma again was described in detail by one participant, Golti, who said,

> I really wasn't fat when I look at my pictures, but my brothers used to tease me about having a big butt, so I would try to watch what I ate and stuff . . . Well, I had mean brothers . . . And my dad was mean too. He used to make fun of me. I'm just big-boned, so even if I lose a lot of weight, I'm not going to be small . . . I came from a very abusive childhood.

She went on to say that she had "big [self] projects" lined up over the next few months because she was not only getting bariatric surgery but also dental surgery. Describing her mother and step-father as "abusive and neglectful," Golti attributed both her current struggles with weight and her cavities and gum loss to the poor diet she received growing up. At the same time, she also pointed out the connections between weight gain and stress later in life, saying that she gained 70 pounds "after my sister elected to stand in front of a train in Texas" a few years previously, and the gained more weight after her nephew, "who my husband and I partly raised," was killed "riding his motorcycle at 100 mph when he was 20 years old."

We also noted that the clinic program's (understandable) orientation around issues relating to weight and health meant that individuals were far more comfortable discussing weight and physical health as motivating factors for opting for bariatric surgery. Patients were far less comfortable discussing aesthetics, body image, and experienced weight-related stigma, including as motivators for surgery. Moreover, there were clear gendered differences in the degree of expressed discomfort: men were far less likely to openly discuss their body ideals, their emotions as they related to eating and food, and their felt vulnerabilities connected to experienced stigma. Todd went so far as to say,

> From what I've seen, most of the women that I have met through the study group or support groups and things like that have done it primarily just to lose the weight, where most of the men I found had done it, like myself, for other medical reasons . . . No, I went through it without it [emotional and social support]. I didn't have anybody really to talk to about it afterwards. I don't know how to describe it. I didn't have it. It was okay. I didn't go looking for it. It was going to be what it was. I made the decision. I knew why I needed to do it. I achieved what I wanted out of it and then some, and then a lot more. But it did what I wanted it to do and it didn't matter what anybody else thought, whether it was positive, negative, or anything else.

Many other men we spoke with did describe receiving, and being grateful for, familial and social support. Nevertheless, Todd's portrayal of himself as pragmatically engaging with surgery as a tool for greater health, and as a man who did not have emotional and aesthetic ties to his physical body, was not uncommon. Additionally, the bariatric program at Mayo Clinic does include a mandatory assessment of emotional state and readiness for surgery by the program's psychologist and male patients tended to express far greater annoyance over this requirement than did female patients.

Issues related to the intersection of weight and other layered discriminations also emerged. Alice, for example, who was very self-contained in the context of the mandatory behavioral changes classes, was far more forthcoming in the interviews.

> When I turned 41, I had put on a little weight. I had put on weight. And I had gotten up to—no, I did get up to—I moved to Tennessee and that's why I can remember. And I was weighing close to 200. And I started to get—that's another thing, appearance. I have this like—everybody has something different, but right here is kind of like fat [pats base of neck] . . . So yes, and I said—I

> thought maybe I was having some kind of neck problem because I worked in a factory. And so I said, "Well, what is that?" And he said, and this was in Tennessee and I'm telling you I got really pissed off, he said, "That's fat. You just love the pork, don't you?" I know, this country Tennessee doctor said this to me and I'm coming from Detroit and I'm thinking, "Boy, you will never get any of my Blue Cross anymore" . . . They [all the doctors who belittled her] were white little country doctors. That sounds racist, but they were now that I think about it, you know? Yeah. And I remember he said that. And my feelings were hurt.

Alice clearly made the connection in her interview that her negative encounters with doctors were a result of being African American and female and obese.

DISCUSSION

We know that literature searches of the kind employed here are not exhaustive. For example, we know that Gimlin's (2002) work on women's body-centered projects explores, in one section, the ways in which members of the National Association to Advance Fat Acceptance (NAAFA) negotiate their status as "fat women." Her book was not visible via either search engine. Other valuable qualitative work emerging from research into bariatric surgery specifically, including research by Groven (Groven et al. 2013a, 2013b, 2013c, 2012, 2010), Natvik (Natvik et al. 2013), Warholm (Warholm et al. 2014), and Christensen (2012) likewise remained invisible.

Such exceptions aside, however, our primary argument—that the perspectives of the real people associated with the pathologized and publicized large bodies are not being systematically explored by anthropologists from an ethnographic perspective—still stands. The result of these gaps is that we perpetuate the invisibility of fat bodies—or at least of their experiences and voices. In so doing, we do not address how the needs of "obese/fat" people can be articulated and then translated into observable differences and tailored to actually be implemented in medical settings.

Our research is already improving our understanding of the role that gender plays in the creation of weight-related stigma, which is difficult to extract from prior ethnographic analyses simply because of small, convenience sampling and a focus on women. We know from work such as Boero's (2012, 2010) that women's navigation of identity changes as weight is lost is very different from that of men in the United States. We also know that experiences involving weight management, attitudes toward body image, social patterns affected by weight and beauty concerns, and deployment of body capital show gendered differences in many instances, with the impact of body and weight concerns disproportionately felt by women (Becker 1995; Bordo 1993; Carpenter et al. 2000; Carryer 1997; Edmonds 2010; Gimlin 2002; Fallon 1990;

Jackson 1992; Millman 1980; Nichter 2000). We are interested, however, in the specific ways in which gendered identities impact experiences relating to weight, weight loss, and bariatric surgery—at a time when increasing numbers of men are feeling increased pressure to conform to body norms but do not appear to be articulating the pressures in the same way that women do.

Based on our own pilot research with patients, there appear to be profound gendered differences in experiences with pre-surgery preparation. This appears especially true with respect to the mandatory requirement that Mayo bariatric patients track their emotional state while eating. The mixed-gender nature of the mandatory pre-operative classes also appears to inhibit frank discussion around body image and stigma experiences. Post-surgery experiences, including expressed need for social support from friends, also appear to have gendered differences and this has implications for long-term tracking and support of post-operative patients.

Moreover, gender and race appear to interact in complicated and as yet poorly understood ways for people attending the Mayo Clinic bariatric program. Within the U.S., significant associations between poverty, racial minority status, female gender, and obesity risk are well-established by population-level analyses and ethnographic studies alike (Belle et al. 2008; Brewis 2011; Casper and Moore 2009; Durkin et al. 1999; Gravlee 2009; Krieger 1999; Martin et al. 2010; McClure 2013; Sudan et al. 2014). Thus, "being fat" intersects with other vulnerable social categories in ways that could either alleviate or compound how stigma is felt. Research on "compounded stigmas" in the context of HIV/AIDS (Obermeyer et al. 2009; Parker et al. 2002) indicates that layered or compounded stigmas mutually reinforce one another. These layers and intersections are rarely unpacked, however, with respect to weight-related stigma (Link and Phelan 2001; Puhl and Heuer 2009). Indeed, racial minority status until recently has all too often been assumed, especially when it coincides with female gender, to counter-balance mainstream US fat stigma, even as studies (e.g., McClure 2013) now increasingly point out that fat stigma has penetrated all communities in the United States today. As a result, bariatric patients register multiple sources of stigma that may or may not interact (e.g., female, African American, and extremely obese), but the focus on obesity and health within the bariatric program—while understandable—appears to de-motivate full engagement from those individuals who are registering more than one type of stigma experience.

CONCLUSION AND RECOMMENDATIONS

As noted, there is arguably no better example of the ways in which multiple anthropological concerns converge at the site of the socially and economically stigmatized, "failed" body project of an obese individual living in the United States' simultaneously obesogenic and fat-stigmatizing environment. Analysis often ends after describing individual obese bodies, obese communities, and risk factors for obesity; thus, the extremely obese body is muted, flattened and rendered two-dimensional under its own weight in much of this writing. By focusing on those most affected by the social and medical meanings of obesity, this study contributes substantively to the goal of moving obesity into its own theoretical space.

Our own research provides one example of the ways in which collaborations between clinicians and ethnographers can push forward our understanding of obesity and the efficacy of medical interventions for people who want to lose weight. Partnering with Mayo Clinic, a globally recognized leader in medical practice innovation and one especially concerned with how to enhance patient experiences, maximizes the chance of useful application and broad dissemination of the study results to improve the non-medical aspects of people's encounters within complex modern health systems. One important recommendation stemming from our research has to do with the need to create programmatic environments that feel welcoming to people from diverse backgrounds, including those who have had negative experiences in clinical settings in the past. Another is that not explicitly addressing issues of difference stemming from gender and race, particularly in group settings (both support groups and classes), is inhibiting discussion and support of individuals' diverse views and lived experiences. Both of these recommendations—based on research gathered from in-depth, longitudinal ethnographic study—have the potential to make solid, observable improvements in clinical care provided to bariatric patients. A clinic-based ethnography designed to assess the efficacy of such changes can, in turn, yield recommendations for "best practices" that may help to improve bariatric care in a much wider range of clinical settings.

Our overarching argument here has been that, despite the proliferating literature on obesity, people living with obesity have received too little attention. There is a clear lack of in-depth, ethnographic research on people classified as obese. There is also a clear lack of clinically-engaged ethnography that aims to *improve* patient experiences for these populations. In this paper, moreover, we also demonstrate how research questions exploring obesity, race, gender, and other problems of intersectionality have been too little examined in research with bariatric patients. Such questions have the potential to add new insights to scholarly research on obesity and to improve the quality of care in clinical settings.

Chapter 11

Fat by Any Other Name[1]

Perceptions of "Obesity" in Clinical Settings

Deborah L. Williams, Alexandra A. Brewis, Sarah S. Trainer, and Jose Rosales Chavez

In the context of applied anthropology, we understand that the selection and deployment of terminology is critically important to how health education, prevention, and intervention efforts play out on the ground, and ultimately their likely level of success. Health messaging, terminology, and related discourse help to shape how we think and feel about issues of health, the body, self, and identity. Thus, the terminology used in public and private settings plays a part in how we perceive ourselves and others, influences our responses and motivations, and may contribute to stigmatization and discrimination. Indeed, disparaging or insensitive language can actually increase unhealthy behaviors or result in avoiding health care all together. Changing the way we talk about health, then, can have powerful impacts. For example, we now know that re-naming conditions such as schizophrenia, borderline personality disorder, and ADHD can reduce associated stigma and improve outcomes for mental health conditions (Hayward and Bright 1997; Levin 2006; Link 1987; Link et al. 1989). Building on this work, we wanted to know if the same concept could be applied to how obesity is perceived and discussed in the United States.

"Fat" and "obese/obesity" are two terms for large bodies that have become prevalent in everyday language in the United States. Rising obesity rates over the last two decades have stimulated a growing public discourse on weight, large bodies, and what is needed to address the "obesity epidemic." "Obese/obesity" is the term used in formal medical and scientific settings, and is also increasingly used in the media and policy debates (Boero 2012; Saguy and Almeling 2007; Hilton et al. 2012; Brewis 2011; Puhl and Heuer 2009; Saguy 2013). "Fat" is, by contrast, a key term used in everyday interpersonal exchanges, such as the "fat talk" that is highly prevalent among youth, especially girls (Taylor 2006; Nichter 2000). Sensitive and effective public health messaging requires that we understand how perceptions and uses of terms like "obese/obesity" or "fat" impact individuals, families, and communities (Brewis 2014).

The "clinical encounter" (defined here as the dynamic interactions and exchanges that take place between health professionals and patients seeking health care) is a key interpersonal site for the deployment of weight-related terminology. While the clinical encounter has been analyzed by anthropologists and sociologists, this examination has primarily been within the context of power dynamics, ideology, and social control (Ferzacca 2000; Foucault 1973; Lilleleht 2002; Shildrick and Price 1998; Waitzkin 1989; Willis and Waddington 2013). Much of the research from outside the social science arena has explored issues of general medical discourse, compliance, and the overall structure of the encounter. There is little research exploring how health providers discuss weight, particularly excess weight, with their patients. Only in the last five or six years have researchers begun to delve into the health care setting to understand some of the factors that may influence successful outcomes.

PREVIOUS WORK

Lewis et al. (2010) used qualitative data derived from interviews with adults with a BMI ≥ 30 to conclude that patients felt strongly that clinical discussions needed to be less about weight itself, and more about general health. In particular, patients felt that practitioners focused on their weight rather than addressing the specific medical complaints that brought them to the provider. Several survey-based studies (e.g., Dutton et al. 2010; Gray et al. 2011; Puhl et al. 2013; 2011; Volger et al. 2012; Wadden and Didie 2003) consistently report that patients with BMIs (CDC 2014, WHO 2014) above "Normal Weight" categories viewed the terms "obese," "fat," and "fatness" as undesirable; these patients did not want such terms used within the clinical encounter. At the same time, other studies (e.g., Baron 2011, Tailor and Ogden 2009) have shown doctors are also often uncomfortable with using the term "obese" when talking with patients. A study in the United Kingdom found that health care students rated use of the term "obesity" negatively, and "fat" or "fatness" even more negatively, and preferred less value-laden terms (Swift et al. 2013). Together these studies have led to some concrete recommendations, including a carefully-worded directive from the National Institute of Health advising healthcare providers to "Use terms preferred by patients, such as 'weight,' 'excess weight,' 'unhealthy body weight,' and 'BMI,' or ask your patient what terms he or she prefers" (NIDDK 2014). A very similar directive was published by Yale University's Rudd Center for

Food Policy and Obesity (2014). There have not been any studies to date on how or if these recommendations have been instituted in practice.

Though we know relatively little about the ways in which "obesity" is used by health professionals in the clinical setting, we know even less about the ways in which lay people use and perceive the term both inside and outside the clinic walls. One of the few such studies (Vartanian 2010) found that university undergraduates showed more negative attitudes toward individuals labeled with the term "obese" than when individuals were labeled "fat." This perhaps indicates the very fact that "obesity" is associated with a clinical setting and makes its use in social interactions more serious than the use of "fat." Of course, deployment of "fat" as a descriptor does have negative repercussions as well, at least in a society with as high rates of weight-related stigma as the mainstream U.S. exhibits today (Brewis 2011; Puhl and Heuer 2009). A different study (Smith et al. 2007), also on a college campus, showed that use of the terms "fat" and "obese" to describe certain individuals to undergraduate students resulted in the participants rating the individuals so labeled as heavier than when other terms were employed. Increased knowledge about how people use and respond to different terminology, both in health care and non-health-care settings, is important to understanding the success, or lack thereof, of public health interventions.

A NEW STUDY

Here, we consider how deployment of terms related to excess weight might affect how young people perceive and react to clinical encounters related to weight. This study focuses on a young population, college students that we have elsewhere shown to be actively engaged in fat talk (Trainer et al. 2015). Weight is an issue on college campuses, both because rising child obesity rates means many students are already overweight by their late teens (Brewis 2011; Murray and Anzeljc 2011; Lavizzo-Mourey 2009), and because weight gain is a common problem across the undergraduate years (Huang et al. 2003).

For the study we discuss in this chapter, we were interested in identifying how a generally healthy, educated sample of students reacted to "obesity," "fat," and related terminology, with a specific focus on the acceptable use of those terms in medical/clinical settings. This information can then be used to improve health services and behaviors on campuses. In our analysis we focused on two key variables that could affect people's reactions: their own body weight and gender. Own body size could be important given that lay terms like "fat" might have more salience for those who believe they themselves fit the category. Second, gender is potentially important given that prior ethnographic studies suggest girls are much more likely than boys to engage in fat talk. Increased use of the term in everyday life could shape its acceptability.

METHODS

Research activities were conducted at Arizona State University (ASU), the largest comprehensive public university in the United States, whose student population matches the socio-demographics of the wider state population. In the context of this study, students were defined as anyone currently enrolled in a university-level course, and all data collection occurred in the spring semester of 2012. Students under 18 years of age were excluded from participation.

For the first stage of the study, we recruited a representative sample of 202 ASU undergraduate students. To derive a representative student sample, we applied what is known as a spatialized and randomized sampling strategy. Research assistants walked randomly selected N-S and E-W transects across campus selecting the *n*th person. A random number from 5 to 10 was selected each day to represent the *n*th person (e.g., if the number was 6, the recruiter would walk along the specified path and count each person passing until she met the sixth student). Each participant was asked to provide five words to describe four different sized silhouettes of each gender, including "thin," "normal," "overweight," and "obese" (medically categorized, WHO 2014), for a total of 40 adjectives describing eight figures. The specific elicitation was: *Here are four silhouettes of male/female university students. Please give us five adjectives (descriptive words) that come to mind when you look at the man's/ woman's body shape number.* Using the responses to the overweight and obese silhouettes, elicited words were then collapsed to take into account word variants (e.g., "obese" and "obesity"). We then rejected any word variant that appeared less than three times. By this procedure we identified 21 weight-related terms known to students at this university, which then formed the basis of the word-term questionnaire we used in the second phase of the study.

For the second phase of this study, we used a purposive sampling technique to identify specific locations on campus and recruit participants, with recruitment conducted outside the health center, dining halls, recreation centers, and residence halls. We recruited 264 participants to complete a survey. Participants were measured for height and weight (to calculate BMI; see WHO 2014), and were also asked about their perceived risk of being obese within their lifetime to elicit if there were response differences between individuals who perceived they themselves might become overweight from those who anticipated a normal weight throughout their lifetime. Out of the total of 264 students, 4.2% were underweight (<18.50 BMI), 66.3% were normal weight (18.50–24.99), 18.9% were overweight (25–29.99), and 8.3% were obese (≥30). There proved to be no significant differences in the demographics (mean weight, mean age, ethnicity, and gender) of students recruited using the systematic sampling strategy in Phase 1 vs. in the purposive sampling strategy in Phase 2. In other words, our sample was an accurate reflection of overall student demographics at ASU.

Our prompt in Phase 2, which presented to students the 21 selected obesity-related terms, was modified from Wadden and Didie's (2003) questionnaire: *Imagine that you are visiting your doctor for a checkup. The nurse has measured your weight and found that you are over your recommended weight. The doctor will be in shortly to speak with you. Doctors can use different terms to describe weight. Please indicate how desirable or undesirable you would find each of the following terms if your doctor used it.* Participants used a five-point Likert-type scale where –2 represented "very undesirable," 0 was "neutral," and 2 was "very desirable." The order of presentation of the 21 key terms within each survey was randomized for each participant and each question. Students also completed an "Attitudes toward Obese Persons" (ATOP) scale and a "Beliefs about Obese People" (BAOP) scale developed to assess people's explicit stigmatizing attitudes to weight (Allison et al. 1991).

Statistical analyses were conducted in SPSS version 21, with final regression models defined and derived in SPSS AMOS version 19. Alpha was set at 0.05. Significant covariates included in our regression analysis were age, exercise levels, female gender, body size (measured BMI), ATOP score, and people's perceptions of their own risk for weight gain. Ethnicity proved to not be significant and was removed from the analysis.

In addition, to contextualize findings, ST conducted in-depth interviews with 15 undergraduate students: ten females and five males of varying weight categories. We repeated the three prompts asked in the original phase 1 survey, but elicited more in-depth, extended responses following these questions, asking students why they responded in the way they did to the survey prompts.

RESULTS

Figure 11.1 shows the participant responses on the desirability of the use in clinical settings of each of the 21 weight-related terms identified in Phase 1. Overall, the least preferred terms were "huge," "fat," and "chubby." "Obese/obesity" was rated negatively overall, but was viewed as more desirable on

Item	*Component 1 Everyday Terms*	*Component 2 Medical Terms*
Heavy	0.767	
Excess weight	0.725	
Excess fat	0.722	
Overweight	0.701	
Big	0.701	
Weight problem	0.699	
Obese/Obesity	0.691	
Large/Large size	0.689	
Hefty	0.687	
Fat/Fatness	0.683	
High BMI	0.653	
Chubby	0.648	
Huge	0.612	
Thick	0.605	
Plump	0.586	
Round	0.585	
Unfit	0.563	
Fluffy	0.485	
Unhealthy BMI		0.655
Unhealthy weight		0.620
BMI		0.547
% of variance explained	41.4%	17.4%

Figure 11.1 Principal Component Analysis for Weight Related Terminology.

average than nine other terms. The students rated technical terms as most preferred: "BMI," "unhealthy weight," "high BMI," and "unhealthy BMI." Scores by weight category (normal weight vs. overweight/obese) and by gender (male vs. female) showed similar distributions. In other words, students rated terms similarly regardless of their own body size or gender.

Using principal component analysis (see Figure 11.2), we found 16 items loaded together onto the first factor that were clearly the less-medical or scientific terms: "huge," "fat," "chubby," "plump," "fluffy," "hefty," "round," "thick," "big," "obese," "heavy," "large/large size," "excess fat," "excess weight," "overweight," and "weight problem." The second factor related to specifically technical terms (and notably excluded "obesity"): "unhealthy BMI," "BMI," and "unhealthy weight." "Unfit" had essentially a neutral score in terms of desirability but sorted with the popular terms in our analysis. These two factors explained 59% of the variation. We then conducted a regression analysis in AMOS using our basic model, specifically predicting which people would find the use of the terms "obese/obesity" undesirable in a clinical setting. Of all the proposed factors, the only significant predictors

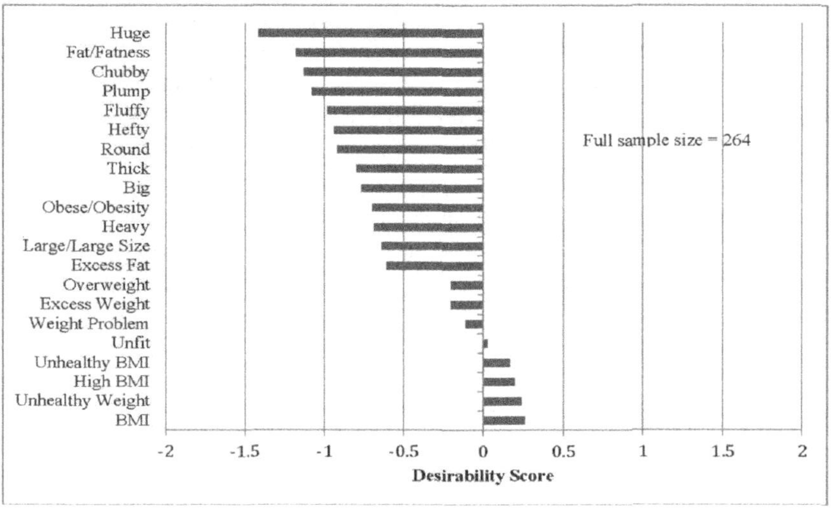

Figure 11.2 Mean participant scores on preference of weight-related terms in clinical settings, assessed on a 5-point Likert-type scale ranging from −2 = "Very Undesirable" to +2 = "Very Desirable".

of perceived undesirability for the term "obesity" were being female and having a higher BMI. For the undesirability of the term "fat," the sole significant predictor was being female ($p < 0.05$).

Among the students who participated in the in-depth interviews, there was universal agreement that in a clinical setting, it is unprofessional and inappropriate for a medical professional to use "fat," "chubby," "chunky," or other "slang words" to talk about larger body size in patients. A health care professional "should use distancing, professional language and rely on the facts of the disease," said one female student, and "there is no reason EVER to use a loaded, hurtful word like 'fat' in a clinical encounter."

A few students (all normal weight and primarily male) felt it would be acceptable for a medical professional to use the term "obese" in a clinical encounter but the majority of the interviewees, especially those who self-categorized as overweight or obese, vehemently disagreed with this. One student who self-described as "extremely fat" remarked that although it would be "unprofessional" for "fat" to be used in a clinical setting, she was equally tired of hearing herself described as "obese" by doctor after doctor. This individual summed up her experiences as "different ways of dressing it up." Another student (male and overweight) commented that although "fat" was not an appropriate descriptor for doctors to use with patients, he felt that "obese" was too pathologizing: "To be obese is to be that person riding a scooter through Walmart in order to buy Cheez-Its," he said.

Alternatively, students suggested that in a clinical setting it is best for a medical professional to frame excess weight in terms of "x pounds needing to be lost," as the preferred approach and to justify raising the issue at all by citing elevated risk for associated diseases. As one female interviewee explained it, "Talking about diseases [associated with obesity] approaches the topic [of weight] kind of sideways, and then you get to avoid fat-shaming . . . There's no reason, really, to even need to use 'fat' or 'obese.'" Others agreed with this, and a number also pointed out (all-too correctly) that the terms themselves can be quite imprecise in how they are used, even in medical settings.

DISCUSSION

Understanding how people react to the language that has developed around the physical state of obesity (Brewis 2011; Puhl and Heuer 2009) is important, for the terminology that we use helps to shape how we think about the conditions the terminology describes. This in turn shapes social stigma vs. acceptance, affects how people perceive their own and others' weight, influences the ways in which individuals respond to medical or public health recommendations, and ultimately impacts the degree to which people are motivated toward health behavior change (Brewis 2014, 2011).

A primary finding here is that university students view "obesity" as a problematic word, even though it remains deployed in health care settings, policy debates, and media. When we examined how the acceptability of different obesity-related terms sorted together in a factor analysis, we found that people were clearly distinguishing terms perceived as technical from those seen as lay (such as "BMI" from "chubby"). Interestingly, "obesity" sorted with neither the technical terms nor the lay terms, though "obesity" and "fat" clustered together. This finding suggests that people do not consider "obesity" as a technical term like "BMI," but neither is it viewed as a term appropriate for casual social conversations. When we examined the range of factors that might shape the acceptability of weight-related terms, we found that despite both genders' overall negative valuation of such terms as "fat," "heavy," or "chubby," women were more likely to use these descriptors in personal conversations. This suggests that while women are aware of the stigmatizing nature of these descriptors, they continue to internalize and operationalize body norms in how they employ terms. Two concerns emerge from this finding: (1) women are more likely to have a negative body-image and engage in self-stigmatization, and (2) stigmatization and discrimination have their own negative health consequences (Sagay 2012, Puhl & Heuer 2010).

The partitioning of preferred terminology between clinical and social settings is reflective of the general trend toward the medicalization of the so-called obesity problem (Saguy 2013). Medicalized or technical language is often assumed to increase the neutrality of a health-associated condition, resulting in a lessening of stigmatization. For example, AIDS was originally stigmatized as a "gay" disease but later redefined through vigorous health campaigns (Pomeranz 2008). Health campaigns can, however, have the reverse effect, as evidenced by health campaigns in the early 1900s that warned that close contact with African Americans would spread tuberculosis (Pomeranz 2008). More recently, anti-smoking campaigns in the United States, though successful in reducing smoking behaviors among Americans, increased negative perceptions not just of smoking itself but also of people who smoked, in effect often vilifying them (Graham 2012). The fact that "obesity" has emerged as a less preferred term in both clinical and social settings may be indicative of the stigmatization not just of obesity but also of obese persons. Thus, a preference for descriptors such as "unhealthy BMI," which is a trait that a person possesses but not necessarily a trait that a person *is* ("you are obese" vs. "you have an unhealthy BMI") makes sense.

Medicalized terminology also pathologizes: it implies a degree of both seriousness and severity (Tailer and Ogden 2009). This might also be responsible for influencing the trends we observed in terminology preferences, toward those that focus on weight in a general context and are de-coupled from "obesity" as a diseased state with implied co-morbidities (Swift et al. 2013). In lay contexts, students may feel that using "obese/obesity" not only increases the stigmatization of the individual based on their body weight but also renders their body diseased. Use of "fat," by contrast, stigmatizes but does not necessarily suggest actual disease or pathology.

Also noteworthy here is that the context-specific deployment of weight-related terminology does not appear to have diminished students' use of stigmatizing language across these contexts, despite awareness of the negative effects of such language. Elsewhere, we have described in more detail how students deploy "fat talk" on this campus (Trainer et al. n.d.); however, overall students found many weight-related terms problematic, particularly "fat" and "obese," though they continue to use these terms in everyday life. These findings suggest shifting frames when discussing weight, without shifting underlying prejudices against larger bodies. For instance, students' preferred terms in the clinical setting are technical, directly related to health, and in general de-personalized, but significantly, the terms are also "actionable" nouns, meaning they indicate a corporeal state (poor health or illness, etc.) that requires action or intervention. We could expect this when defining excess weight as a medical problem (and indeed this is one of the underlying goals of defining obesity medically). Contrast this to the descriptive terms students view as acceptable within their casual social interactions, especially use of the word "fat." This terminology was personalized, descriptive (adjectives), and often emotionally loaded. This suggests that students (consciously or unconsciously) use a moralistic frame to view excess weight as a personal characteristic or defect rather than a state of being or health. This type of framing is consistent with stigmatization and suggests that while large body size is reframed as a medical condition in clinical settings, outside these settings students continue to view overweight and obesity through a moralistic lens.

SUGGESTIONS FOR INTERVENTIONS AND CONCLUSION

What are the implications of these findings with respect to interventions, especially those aimed at young people? In clinical environments, the use of technical language is a mixed bag for patients, on the one hand reinforcing perceptions of medical expertise (and authority) while increasing patient anxiety, potentially reducing the patient's perception of self-efficacy and control, and increasing self-blame (Tailor and Ogden 2009). Disparaging or emotionally charged terms can be counterproductive to patient motivation, and there is some indication that insensitive language or communication styles actually increase unhealthy behaviors (Puhl et al. 2013; Gray et al. 2011).

Health professionals need to take into account patients' preferred terms in discussing weight and weight-related health issues. This is particularly important with college students as they take charge of their own health and learn how to navigate the health care system and patient-provider relationships. Health in the context of young adulthood is often assumed, particularly by young adults. Initial self-initiated health encounters can therefore be disconcerting and stressful. Tailoring terminology and practice to this age group is crucial in establishing good patient engagement and fostering successful treatment.

Early and frequent education of health providers is one way to bring a change to the clinical encounter. For example, physicians, nurse practitioners, and physician assistants complete a physical diagnosis course (which includes how to take a patient history) before their clinical training. This type of course should address how to discuss sensitive topics with patients to ensure good quality care and patient engagement. Training in age and gender-specific body ideals also needs to be addressed. This is particularly important in young adults, who undergo enormous stressors in building identity and self-worth during this life-stage. Discussing weight with this group needs to be conducted in a sensitive and positive manner that supports the dignity of the individual. Given that our data suggests that young women in particular internalize weight-related talk, providers need to be especially aware of how this group experiences weight-related terminology in practice.

In addition, continuing education modules (required for accreditation and licensing) should include discussions on effective health counseling and how to avoid stigmatizing patients, and ultimately sabotaging patient compliance. One way providers could address this is to modify their patient intake forms to include a question asking if patients are comfortable with their current weight. The provider can then adjust the conversation (and language) in response. Additionally, emphasis should be placed on health rather than on ideal body weight and providers given tools and specific prompts to elicit patient concerns. In other words, health care professionals must personalize the patient encounter and actually enquire what terms with respect to body size patients are most comfortable with, rather than relying on one-size-fits-all (literally) approaches, no matter how well-intended.

Finally, effective health messaging needs to take into account audience response. Our findings indicate that terminology is a key component in health messaging about weight. Moreover, the findings suggest that *how* terminology is used impacts audience perceptions. At the population level, this means avoiding stigmatizing language and using terminology and messaging that not only promote awareness but also spur personal action and behavior change. One of the ways we address this at our university is to frame student health interventions within the larger context of engagement, activity, and wellness. A recent university-wide initiative to promote student health provides an example. The initiative is framed as "active engagement"—in a student's own personal health, in university educational and social activities, and in career development. Weight, nutrition, and activity are considered to be part of a larger endeavor that acknowledges health as a process that includes all of these aspects to be important components of health. Technological tools that allow students to track and monitor their activity, nutrition, and weight are available on campus and through the students' personalized university webpages. University activities, services, and outreach are also visible on these pages and integrated within a larger message of the "active student."

The negative connotations associated with the use of "obese/obesity," "fat," and most other descriptors of excess weight or large body size is its own important health message. Given the need to adequately address obesity, and the widespread problem of weight bias, finding a sensitive and acceptable way to talk about weight is crucial to effective treatment. The possible repercussions of negatively-viewed terminology and stigmatization impact the potential success of health campaigns and interventions.

NOTE

1. This study was conducted as part of the ASU-Mayo Clinic Obesity Solutions initiative, with support of the Virginia G. Piper Charitable Trust. We thank the ASU global health students who recruited and conducted the interviews with their peers for this study, and Amber Wutich and Christopher Roberts for the work they contributed in developing the random sampling strategy used in Phase 1. We also thank Erika Jermé for her editing support.

Chapter 12

Obesity as Public Policy

Creating and Changing the Obesogenic Environment

Merrill Eisenberg

Obesity in the United States is a modern day health issue that lends itself well to critical analysis. The industrial food and transportation industries and the policies that support them have created an environment that steers human behavior toward lifestyle choices that promote obesity. But the story is far more nuanced than the pursuit of capitalistic interests at the expense of the health of the masses. Some of the other factors that promote obesity include broader social and economic realities that impact lifestyle (why do we eat so much fast food?), the unintended consequences of public health and sanitation efforts that separated residential, agricultural, industrial, and commercial areas (why do we have to drive to get anywhere we need to go?), and outdated concepts of community that restrict agricultural activity to rural areas (if I can have a dog in the City, why can't I have a chicken?).

Curbing the obesity epidemic is no easy task. There is no one thing that can be done to alter the ecology of daily life to make it easier for people to choose a healthy lifestyle. Federal policy can address the practices of industrialized food production and can counter industry advertising of junk food with public education campaigns, but much of what is making us fat is embedded in the structure of our communities and in the circumstances of our everyday lives. These factors are governed at the community level by policies made in our schools, workplaces, and local governments. While influencing federal policy requires national-level effort and coordination, changing local policy is something that people can do at the community level. However, as the example provided in this chapter will show, it is not always easy and requires knowledge and skills that are not usually available to most citizens, as well as a large dose of patience.

The policy process is a social endeavor that has been described as a "dance" (Redman 1973) that engages many actors with varying agendas, and is far more complicated than what we might have learned in middle school about "how a bill becomes a law." Applied social scientists are well positioned to analyze the local culture of policy making, to use that information to build a community effort to make change, and to provide reliable data to inform the process. Working collaboratively with community members, policy makers, regulators, and professional staff, applied social scientists can play a significant role in creating a community environment that supports healthy eating and active living.

This chapter will begin with a summary of the current obesity situation in the U.S. and a discussion of why obesity is a serious concern for American society. An ecological model of body weight will be presented and the policies that have created an obesogenic environment will be described, focusing first on physical activity and then on food consumption. The public health response to obesity, focusing on environmental, systems and policy approaches, will be described, followed by an ethnographic account of how one community has taken steps to amend the zoning code to systematically support healthy food availability at the neighborhood level. A description of the Multiple Streams theory of policy development is provided and is used as a framework for understanding what transpired and lessons learned.

THE PROBLEM

Americans are growing fatter. Back in the late 1970s, 14.5% of adults had a Body Mass Index of 30 or higher, and were therefore considered to be obese (Flagel 1998). By 2013, the prevalence of obesity among U.S. adults had risen to 34.9% (Ogden 2014). U.S. females have consistently been more likely to be obese than males, and African Americans and Hispanics have been more likely to be obese than Whites, but the prevalence rate of adult obesity has increased for all population groups. The prevalence of childhood obesity (defined as above the 95th percentile for children of the same age and sex) has also increased over the years, following the same race/ethnicity and gender pattern as the adult prevalence rate, though since 2003 it has stabilized at 16.9% (Ogden 2014).

Obesity is an underlying cause of many chronic diseases, including heart disease, type 2 diabetes, endometrial, breast and colon cancer, hypertension, cholesterol issues, stroke, liver and gallbladder disease, sleep apnea and respiratory problems, osteoarthritis, and gynecological problems such as abnormal menses and infertility (CDC 2014a). Prevalence of these obesity-related diseases is very high—just about every family in America is touched by at least one of these health conditions. In addition to being a problem of personal and family concern, the increase in obesity is a significant public policy concern as it influences health care costs (Finkelstein 2009), economic productivity (Lehnert et al. 2013), and military readiness (Christeson et al. 2012) for all Americans.

AN ECOLOGICAL MODEL OF BODY WEIGHT

The biology of body weight is a complicated topic that is not entirely understood. Genetic inheritance is a risk factor, and in some cases obesity is the result of other illnesses or medications. However, what and how much we eat, and how much energy we expend play a large role for most individuals. These factors are related to lifestyle; they are malleable and therefore can be subject to intervention.

When lifestyle variables are viewed as a matter of personal choice, the cause for the rise in obesity over the past 40 years is attributed to individuals making poor lifestyle choices. However, lifestyle choices are greatly influenced by the community environment. The type of food that is available and affordable influences what we eat, and the structure of the physical and built environments influences how much energy we expend. Other lifestyle variables, like stress, time availability, discretionary income, culture, and social support also impact the personal choices we make. Many of these variables are outside of personal control.

An ecological approach (Kottak 1999) to body weight is a helpful lens for understanding why Americans are growing fatter and what we can do about it. Figure 12.1 shows an ecological model of body weight, indicating some of the individual, daily environmental and social context, large-scale systems, and public policy level factors that influence diet and physical activity. Starting at the individual level, each level is impacted by those above it. Taken together, they describe what is referred to as an "obesogenic environment" (Swinburn et al. 1999). In order to better understand and address obesity in the United States it is important to take into account all levels of the ecological model.

Systems and Policies That Promote Sedentary Lifestyle

One characteristic of the obesogenic environment is that it promotes a sedentary lifestyle, which is a strong predictor of obesity (Proper et al. 2011). The U.S. Centers for Disease Control and Prevention (CDC 2014b) recommend that in order to maintain health, adults should engage in 2.5 hours of

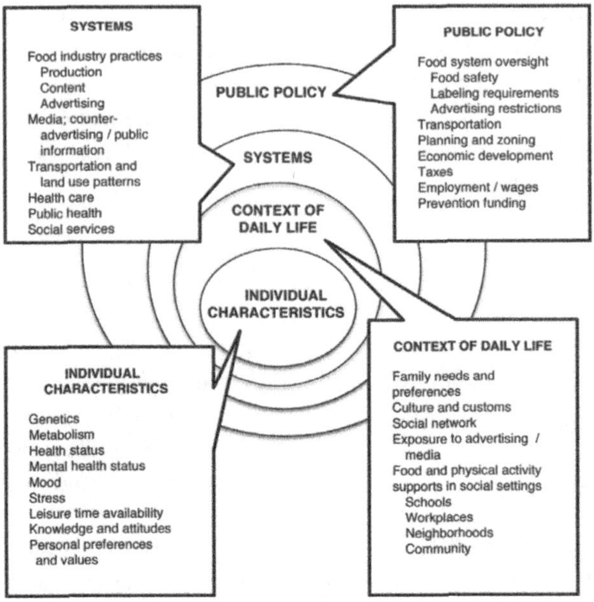

Figure 12.1 An Ecology of Body Weight.

moderate-intensity aerobic activity (such as brisk walking) per week, coupled with muscle strengthening activities that work all major muscle groups (hips, legs, back, abdomen, chest, shoulders, and arms) on two or more days per week, or the equivalent. Prior to the twentieth century, physical activity was built into everyday life. Household activities, job-related activities, and getting from one place to another all required individuals to expend greater energy than these tasks typically require today. It was not as necessary to set aside time for exercise. However, twentieth century changes in the structure and geography of our communities, as well as the mechanization of many jobs, have reduced the amount of physical activity required for everyday life and have relegated physical activity to a recreational activity.

The widespread American adoption of the automobile in the early twentieth century was a harbinger of the obesity epidemic, leading to the replacement of a system of electric streetcars and trollies with diesel engine bus systems in American cities. Because buses were less desirable to riders and less profitable to operators (St. Clair 1981), ridership and profits declined, and public transportation systems across America waned as the reliance on the individual automobile increased. Whether or not the decisions to rip up trolley tracks in favor of buses was part of a conspiracy by General Motors and other combustion engine companies to destroy the public transportation system in order to increase public demand for automobiles remains a matter of debate (Snell 1974; St. Clair 1981). Regardless of the intention, the result made a major contribution to the creation of an obesogenic environment.

The increase in reliance on individual automobile travel coincided with and was supported by land use and urban development policies of the early twentieth century that were established to protect public health. During the late nineteenth and early twentieth centuries, U.S. cities were plagued with industrial pollution and manure from horses that were the main form of transport. In response to these sanitary and public health problems, municipalities adopted zoning regulations to separate residential, commercial, industrial, and agricultural activities (Schilling and Linton 2005; Birch and Silver 2009). The separation of land uses by zone required people to travel greater distances in their daily lives, a need that was fulfilled by the automobile. It is ironic that the 1926 landmark Supreme Court decision, *Ambler Realty v The Village of Euclid*, which legalized local exclusionary zoning ordinances using a public health rationale, has led to the proliferation of urban sprawl, the "geography of nowhere" (Kunstler 1993), and an environment that is detrimental to public health because it promotes obesity by making it necessary to drive, rather than walk, in order to conduct most daily activities.

Other characteristics of the built environment that promote obesity and are determined by transportation, land use and urban design policies include the density of residential, employment, and institutional uses, a non-grid approach to street design, and the lack of sidewalks, setbacks, and traffic calming features such as speed bumps and traffic circles (Feng et al. 2010). At the neighborhood level, variables that are related to low levels of physical activity include neighborhood safety issues (Burdette et al. 2006; Evensen et al. 2012), and proximity to recreation facilities (Humple et al. 2003). It is no wonder that zip code has been found to be a stronger predictor of obesity than either individual income or race/ethnicity (Drewnowski et al. 2009).

The twentieth century also brought significant changes to the food system that have resulted in a high calorie, low nutrient diet for many Americans. We have seen a sharp increase in consumption of processed refined grains and sugars, refined vegetable oils, salt, and fatty meats. This diet is part of the etiology of many obesity-related chronic diseases (Cordain et al. 2005), and is the result of the industrialization of the food system that occurred during the nineteenth and twentieth centuries.

Food production had become industrialized by the end of the nineteenth century in response to increasing urbanization (Deutsch 2012), and the ingredients used and manufacturing practices that were implemented were meant to maximize corporate profits, rather than to maximize health. The journey of food from the field to the fork now included many new opportunities for spoilage, infestation with bugs and animal droppings, and adulteration with chemicals, preservatives, and dyes. Federal oversight of the food system began in 1906 with the passage of the Pure Food and Drug Act and the Federal Meat Inspection Act. Sanitation issues improved, but nutritional composition was not addressed. Further, federal farm subsidies that began during the Hoover administration were expanded in the early 1970s to foods that are directly linked to obesity (Walinga 2014). For example, subsidies for corn production began in the early 1970s (Glauber 2013), providing an incentive for corn growers to develop new uses for their product. High fructose corn syrup is one such use. The 1000% increase in the consumption of high fructose corn syrup that occurred between 1970 and 1990 is linked to the rise in obesity (Bray et al. 2003).

Between 1970 and 2013, consumption of meals eaten away from home also increased—from 25.9% to 43.1%—a change that is attributed to systems and policy issues including more women in the workforce, an increase in incomes, the low cost and high availability of fast food outlets, and increased advertising and promotion of fast food (USDA 2014a). Meals consumed away from home are higher in calories and are of poorer nutritional quality than meals consumed at home (Lin et al. 2004; Boumtje et al. 2005; Bowman et al. 2004). Further, high calorie fast food is less expensive than healthier choices that are on the menu. For example, at McDonalds you can fill up on Chicken McNuggets (940 calories) for $1 but the Premier Southwest Salad with Grilled Chicken (290 calories) costs $4.79 (McDonalds 2014)—the salad is 15.5 times more expensive per calorie than the Chicken McNuggets.

The industry practice of "supersizing," especially prominent since the 1980s, has significantly increased portion sizes and calorie intake (Young and Nestle 2002). For example, a typical cheeseburger contained 333 calories 20 years ago, but now contains 590 calories, a 77% increase (NHLB 2013). The availability of cheap, high calorie fast food at the neighborhood level is related to obesity prevalence (Fraser et al. 2010), and the density of fast food outlets is highest in low income/minority neighborhoods (Fleischhacker 2011), where obesity is most prominent.

Food industry advertising and branding practices, which create an environment filled with messages that influence food choices, have also been identified as a factor contributing to the obesity epidemic (Chandon and Wansink 2010). The Rudd Center reports that in 2012, ". . . fast food restaurants spent $4.6 billion in total on all advertising, an 8% increase over 2009. For context, the biggest advertiser, McDonald's, spent 2.7 times as much to advertise its products ($972 million) as all fruit, vegetable, bottled water, and milk advertisers combined ($367 million)" (Rudd Center 2013, 30). Advertising and branding that targets children is of special concern, and exposure to food advertisements on television is associated with childhood obesity (McGinnis et al. 2006; Graf et al. 2012). Other research has demonstrated that food industry advertisement disproportionately targets African Americans, a population with high obesity levels (Grier and Kumanyika 2008).

Policy regulating food advertising practices falls under the jurisdiction of the U.S. Federal Trade Commission (USFTC), which collected baseline data on food advertising targeting children and youth in 2008 (McGinnis et al. 2008). In response to the 2008 study the Council of Better Business Bureaus launched the Children's Food and Beverage Advertising Initiative, a voluntary industry self-regulating program to either limit child-directed advertising to foods that meet meaningful uniform nutrition criteria, or to not engage in advertising food products to children at all. Seventeen major food corporations have agreed to follow the child-directed advertising restrictions, including Burger King, McDonald's, Campbell Soup, Dannon, Kellogg, Kraft, Coca-Cola, PepsiCo, and others (Better Business Bureau 2014). A follow-up study in 2012 found "modest improvements" in the nutritional quality of foods marketed to children (USFTC 2012, ES2) and although progress is still needed, the USFTC continues to support self-regulation as opposed to governmental oversight (USFTC 2012, 115).

Public Health and the Ecological Model of Body Weight

The systems and policy issues in the ecology of obesity demonstrate that intervention focused on individuals' choices will not be sufficient to curb the obesity epidemic. Therefore, in addition to individual level interventions such as nutrition education and promotion of physical activity, the U.S. public health community provides advice and funding for obesity prevention efforts at the social context, systems, and policy levels of the ecological model. For example, the American Public Health Association (APHA 2014) has adopted policy statements for addressing obesity that support taxing sugar sweetened beverages (#20122), increasing access to natural environments (#20137), creating a healthy, sustainable food system (#200712), adopting land use and transportation practices (#20099), and framing of food availability and affordability as an environmental justice issue (#20073). Similarly, the CDC recommends strategies that promote the availability of affordable healthy food and beverages, create safe communities that support physical activities, and encourage community members to organize for community change (Keener et al. 2009). The CDC's Division of Community Health provides resources to states, tribes, and local communities for these recommendations through grant programs such as Pioneering Healthy Communities (PHC), Racial and Ethnic Approaches to Community Health (REACH), Communities Putting Prevention to Work (CPPW), and

Partnerships to Improve Community Health (PICH). The purpose of these grants is ". . . to make healthy living easier where people live, work, learn, and play" (CDC 2014c).

What follows is an example of how CPPW dollars were used to combat obesity through policy and systems change at the community level. In 2010, the Pima County (Arizona) Health Department (PCHD) received a $15.75 million grant from the CDC's CPPW program to address obesity prevention through policy, systems, and environmental change. PCHD contracted with local non-governmental organizations to create four place-based teams that focused in neighborhood, schools and childcare settings, worksites, and faith-based organizations. Four additional support teams were created to focus on the food system, the built environment, media, and public policy. The Policy Team, which was situated in the University of Arizona Zuckerman College of Public Health and was directed by this author (an applied anthropologist), was tasked with responding to policy questions raised by the other teams, identifying issues for policy change, educating policy makers and the community about obesity as a policy issue, and building a constituency for public policies that promote healthy lifestyles. Activate Tucson, a community coalition for healthy eating and active living that had been created through a prior PHC grant to the local YMCA in 2005, coordinated communication and collaboration among the eight teams. The CPPW grant period was two years, though because of delays in the contracting process, the community partners were funded for only 20 months.

The remainder of this chapter will focus on just one of the initiatives undertaken by the Pima County project—increasing access to healthy food by removing barriers to urban food production at the home and neighborhood levels. This initiative sought to address the policy level of the ecological model of obesity, and utilized the "multiple streams framework" of policy development (Kingdon 2003), adapted for local level action (Eisenberg 2011) to structure policy research and action activities. As the following ethnographic account of activities demonstrates, CPPW efforts to address the barriers to local level food production required us to augment our focus on obesity with a broader understanding of the community politics of local food production. The constituency for these efforts included not only stakeholders with an interest in health and obesity, but also those who have interests in the environment, the carbon footprint of our food supply and the development of a local economy, as well as those who are engaged in producing food for personal consumption and those who are interested in making local food production their business. Addressing barriers to local food production also required us to focus on very specific aspects of public policy far removed from the "big picture" of the obesity epidemic—the particulars of zoning rules that govern agricultural activity.

ETHNOGRAPHY OF POLICY CHANGE IN PIMA COUNTY, ARIZONA

Pima County, Arizona is located in the Sonoran desert, and shares a 132-mile border with Mexico. At 9,189 square miles, Pima County is about the size of the state of New Hampshire; 85% of the land is federal, state, or tribally owned. There are 23 U.S. Census Designated Places and 15 USDA-designated Colonias in Pima County. The population of just under 1 million is highly concentrated in the eastern portion of the County that contains the City of Tucson and four surrounding small municipalities. At the time the CPPW grant was written the County population was 55.3% White, non-Hispanic and 34.6% Hispanic. Each other racial group constituted less than 4% of the population (US Census Bureau 2010a). Within Tucson, the proportion of Whites was lower and the proportion of every other racial/ethnic group was higher (US Census Bureau 2010b).

The Obesogenic Environment in the Greater Tucson Area

The Sonoran Institute, a nonprofit organization that seeks to encourage community development throughout the American West in a manner respectful of the land and people (Sonoran Institute 2014), provides a concise description of the how the Tucson area has developed over time (see Text Box 12.1).

Text Box 12.1 History of Development in the Tucson Area

Tucson is one of the longest continuously inhabited communities in North America. The ancestors of the Tohono O'odham settled here permanently at least three thousand years ago. In the 1900s, development in Tucson—like that in many western U.S. cities—was a product of our nation's westward expansion, driven by cheap and abundant land. The expansion of railroad lines, especially the Southern Pacific and the Santa Fe, and the introduction of the automobile pushed Tucson's population over twenty thousand following World War I. The city expanded once again during World War II as Davis-Monthan Municipal Airfield became a military airbase. Most of the early growth in Tucson spread eastward, taking advantage of easily developed valley land offering views of the Catalina Mountains. Once development came up against publicly owned lands, it changed direction, heading northwest of the city. Through the 1990s and into this century, development has continued to follow a similar pattern, extending into areas beyond the metropolitan fringe where land remains cheap and accessible and homes on large lots are relatively affordable.

Source: The Sonoran Institute. Building From the Best of Tucson. http://www.sonoraninstitute.org/component/docman/doc_view/1281-building-from-the-best-of-tucson-book-04012002.html

Many current characteristics of the Tucson area exemplify an environment. The public transportation system provides some service, but streets are clogged with traffic. Long commutes for employment and commercial activity are common. The neighborhood environment discourages walking because many neighborhoods have no sidewalks or streetlights. Further, speeding on residential streets is common because the streets are wide. Interview and observational data reveal that few children ride bicycles or walk to school, a situation that is fueled by parents' perceptions of neighborhood safety dangers as well as the decline in neighborhood school attendance, seen locally as a result of open enrollment options, the closing of some neighborhood schools, and the emergence of charter schools.

The lack of availability of affordable healthy food is another obesogenic feature of Pima County, especially for populations at highest risk for obesity. Many geographic areas are defined as "food deserts"—". . . urban neighborhoods and rural towns without ready access to fresh, healthy, and affordable food" (USDA 2014b). Even within the City of Tucson, there are large swaths of geography where there are no grocery stores, although fast food restaurants are abundant. Neighborhoods in the Tucson metropolitan area have been ranked according to a Stress Index that takes into account 27 indicators based on data in the 2000 Census. These include items related to population age, race/ethnicity, disability, poverty, educational attainment, employment status, working mothers and female head of household, crowding, housing age, presence of plumbing, phone, kitchen facilities and access to vehicles (City of Tucson 2014). According to PCHD (Martin 2008), only 6% of supermarkets were located in high or medium-high Stress Index areas, 35% were located in medium Stress Index areas, and 55% were located in low Stress Index areas. Economic development efforts to attract grocery stores to high stress areas have been unsuccessful.

DEVELOPING POLICY TO INCREASE ACCESS TO HEALTHY FOOD: A CHRONOLOGY OF EVENTS AND ACTIVITIES

Southern Arizona has a climate that supports a year-round growing season, so one approach CPPW took to increasing access to healthy food for people living in food deserts was to encourage and support food production in backyards and neighborhoods. Starting in the fall of 2010, the Food Systems team launched projects to expand its backyard and container gardening cooperative in high-risk neighborhoods, and worked with schools to establish school gardens. A local non-profit organization, Community Gardens of Tucson, was engaged to work with neighborhood groups to develop community gardens, and the Built Environment, Schools/Child Care, and Neighborhoods Teams worked at the grassroots to encourage participation and to engage local individuals in planning work for environmental changes that support physical activity and food production projects. Almost immediately the Policy Team received inquiries from those working at the grassroots to clarify the rules for local food production and distribution.

The Policy Team conducted extensive research in winter/spring 2010–11 to identify the rules and regulations around local food production and distribution in Pima County and the five municipalities in eastern Pima County. Policies at the federal, state, county, and municipal level were fully examined and the Team developed a series of Fact Sheets that compiled the rules from the various sources and presented them in easy to read English and Spanish for each jurisdiction. The Team found that most of the restrictions on local food production and distribution are found in municipal and county zoning regulations. The legal process for amending the zoning code in the City of Tucson was also identified. This process included development of draft language by Tucson City zoning staff, a public hearing at the Planning Commission, a recommendation by the Planning Commission, revision of the draft by City staff if necessary, a second public hearing with Mayor and Council, and finally approval by Mayor and Council. Other jurisdictions had similar processes.

Zoning codes are quite complicated and difficult for lay people to interpret. Therefore, in spring of 2011, local zoning officials were asked to review the fact sheets for accuracy. Many zoning officials were surprised to see how their regulations restrict local food production. Pima County zoning officials decided to simply stop enforcing the restriction on selling home garden products from residential properties.

Coincidentally, Tucson was undergoing a Sustainable Code Revision project to develop code amendments that address sustainability issues, including solar energy, alternative fuel installations, and water harvesting. Food production was also part of the Sustainable Code project, but was a lower priority for City staff than the other issues. Staff did not expect that food production would be addressed in the package of sustainable zoning code amendments that they planned to develop. The City had contracted with a national land use and real estate consulting firm, Clarion Associates, to review the existing zoning code and make recommendations for changes to address sustainability issues. When presented with the Fact Sheets describing Tucson's rules related to agriculture, City staff saw an opportunity to make progress on the urban food production component of the Sustainable Code as well and invited the Policy Team to provide input. Other jurisdictions reported that they were waiting for Tucson to complete its sustainability review and revisions so that they could develop compatible rules. Specific barriers to local food production and distribution in urban areas that were found in the Tucson code are shown in Text Box 12.2.

Text Box 12.2 Tucson Urban Agriculture Zoning Restrictions

- Home gardens are permitted but community gardens are not recognized and therefore require a special administrative procedure.
- Sale of food produced in home or community garden settings is prohibited from urban residential properties.
- Farmers' markets are categorized as "swap meets" and are permitted only in Industrial zones. A zoning appeal, which is costly and time consuming, is required for farmers' markets in other zones.
- Neighbors who produce food are prohibited from pooling their products and selling them in neighborhood settings such as schools and churches.
- Keeping animals for food production purposes is restricted to suburban and rural zones and requires 50' property line setbacks for animal shelters.

Source: The City of Tucson, AZ. 1995. Chapter 23 of Tucson Code: Land Use Code. https://www.tucsonaz.gov/files/pdsd/codes-ordinances/Complete_LUC_Sept2012.pdf

While the Tucson code restricts most agricultural activity in urban areas, the teams working in neighborhoods and schools reported a great deal of local food production and distribution activity at the neighborhood level. In particular, many residents had gardens and were engaged in selling produce from their homes. Keeping chickens for food production was believed to be quite common. Typical urban single-family residential lots in Tucson are about 8000 square feet, providing generous yard space for these activities.

People were not knowingly breaking the rules—they were unaware that any rules existed. Since zoning code violations are enforced upon complaint from a neighbor, most people engaged in urban agricultural had been free to break the rules for many years. However, if a neighbor did complain, the activity would have to cease. Relationships between neighbors are sometimes contentious, and reporting a chicken violation is one way neighbors retaliated against each other.

Tucson zoning officials asked the Policy Team to review and comment on interim reports from Clarion Associates, and to develop additional information about animal keeping practices to inform the Sustainable Code amendment process. Their stated goal was that the new code would reflect current practice to the greatest degree possible, while respecting the concerns of neighboring property owners. In the interim, they also agreed to consider keeping backyard chickens as a routine household activity that is permitted on urban residential properties, provided rules for the placement of coops are followed. However, since most urban residential properties are only about 60 feet wide, it remained illegal to keep chickens because it was impossible to observe the 50' property line setback requirements for coops. Zoning staff then agreed to apply a "dog house exemption" to small coops (up to 10 square feet), thus permitting them on the property line. Larger coops were still required to have the 50' setback.

Over the summer and into the fall of 2011, the Policy Team worked closely with zoning officials and the other CPPW Teams to provide information to inform the development of a reasonable zoning code for animal keeping and other urban agriculture activities. Masters level students in Public Health and this author conducted interviews and site visits with people keeping chickens and found that chickens were not the only animals being kept for food purposes. Many food producers kept a complement of animals that included some combination of chickens, goats, rabbits, guinea pigs, and ducks, raising the question of how to determine a total number of animals to be permitted on an urban residential lot. The placement of coops and other animal shelters on property lines, utilizing pre-existing walls or fences as one side of the shelter was also documented. Aerial photos obtained from Google Earth demonstrated the proximity of these shelters to neighboring residences. The number and type of complaints about farm animals received by police and Pima County Animal Control was also documented and found to be rare.

Secondary research was conducted to identify zoning policies related to urban agriculture in other communities. To document potential barriers, we interviewed officials in communities that are permissive with regard to animals. The Team reviewed recommendations for urban agriculture zoning made by the American Planning Association (Mukherji and Morales 2010) and provided a written public health rationale for the urban agriculture code amendments. This was needed to allow the City to override a state law protecting property owners from undue restriction on how they use their property.

In the fall of 2011, the Policy Team made recommendations for re-structuring the Tucson zoning code to recognize urban agriculture and to create definitions of urban agriculture and small farm animals. An "Urban Animal Unit" approach was recommended for determining the number of animals that could be kept. Each type of animal was assigned a unit weight based on its impact on the environment, considering space requirements, waste, and noise. Three scenarios were proposed for establishing the number of units permitted on any property—establishing limits by zone, by property size, and by property size with a cap. The recommendations included permitting animal shelters on property lines provided they are 20' from a neighboring residential structure.

Clarion Associates, a national land-use and real estate consulting firm that had contracted with the City to revamp the zoning code in order to address sustainability issues, also made draft recommendations for urban agriculture. In the ensuing months, the Policy Team worked with City staff to review and comment on animal-related portions of Clarion's recommendations and to continue to provide information about local practice and what other jurisdictions do. The CPPW grant period ended in March of 2012, but the Policy Team leader vowed to continue to participate in the process until the code was changed. Throughout 2012 she convened meetings, made presentations and conducted workshops about the benefits of urban agriculture and zoning barriers to local food production. Audiences included community groups at the ward and neighborhood levels, nonprofit organizations, health care professionals, the municipal water authority, the Mayor and individual City Councilmembers and their staff, the Planning Commission, the Pima Association of Governments, and many others. A Facebook-based stakeholder group, the Tucson City Living Urban Chicken Keeping Society (Tucson CLUCKS), was created to provide the Policy Team leader with a way to communicate with people who keep animals for food production. CLUCKS served as a source of information about animal keeping practices and experiences, and as a vehicle to inform the animal-keeping community about current policy and engaged in the policy process. As of this writing in 2015, almost 2000 people have joined CLUCKS.

By late 2012 the City's contract with Clarion Associates ended. Clarion's recommendations for urban agriculture included many of the recommendations that had been made by the Policy Team, including the Urban Animal Unit approach. However, city staff felt there was a need for additional community input. In March 2013 City staff invited community stakeholders, including the former Policy Team leader, to participate in a Sustainable Code Advisory Committee. The committee consisted of 15 community members with expertise in sustainability issues, including four people knowledgeable about urban food production. Food production was the first topic addressed. The Advisory Committee drafted a zoning code amendment for urban agriculture that included virtually all of the recommendations about animals that had been made by the Policy Team. This draft was released to the public in the summer of 2013.

The release of the draft code amendment was followed by a scathing critique from a small but vocal subset of neighborhood association presidents, calling themselves the "Neighborhood Infill Coalition" and known by City staff to have actively opposed many other zoning proposals. These individuals had been invited to participate on the Sustainable Code Committee, but they had declined. When the Committee released draft Code amendments to the public, these association presidents strongly opposed them and demanded a second community process to revise them. Although their opposition spanned all aspects of the proposed code revision, including community gardens, sale of produce from where it was grown, and farmers, markets, the group was particularly concerned about keeping animals in residential neighborhoods, citing increased risk of bird flu, the potential of attracting wild predators such as hawks, coyotes and javelina to residential areas, and animal welfare concerns.

Wanting to avoid public confrontation over the amendments, City staff accommodated this demand by initiating a second community input process. Four association presidents and four members of the Sustainable Code Committee were appointed to serve on an Urban Agriculture Task Force in the fall of 2013. The meetings were open to other community members, and participation was strong. The Task Force toiled throughout the fall and winter of 2013–2014 to address the concerns voiced by three of the presidents, with virtually no progress. Recognizing an impasse, zoning staff removed the Urban Animal Unit in favor of permitting three small animals plus eight chickens as a compromise with the opposition. The Task Force was disbanded in February 2014 in favor of a series of four open community meetings to provide an opportunity for citizens to voice their opinions.

Public meetings to acquire additional community input were held in May, June, July and October of 2014. The three opposing neighborhood association presidents had predicted that hundreds of people would come out to voice their opposition to urban agriculture at the community meetings. However, there were no public comments, either at the meetings or provided via phone or email, that opposed the amendments based on the concerns of the three neighborhood association presidents. During this time period we learned that the topic of urban agriculture had either not been addressed or had been supported in the three opposing presidents' association meetings. There was no indication that these presidents were speaking for the neighbors they had claimed to represent.

Nevertheless, the first three public meetings did prove to be quite controversial. While much time and energy had been devoted to educating the urban agriculture community about the code amendment project, many local food producers vehemently opposed the new regulations. Much of the opposition was based on the misinformed opinion that the new code language created new barriers to urban food production.

> What the city appears to be trying to do is regulate things that have not previously been regulated. So it seems like we're moving from a position where if it's not explicitly prohibited, it's permitted, to the opposite, where if it's not explicitly permitted, it's prohibited. And I think that's completely un-American.

> I think if I want to support my family and this form of support creates happiness, then why regulate my constitutional right in my pursuit of happiness?

Deep distrust of any government action was a significant barrier to efforts to educate these people about the current rules and how the new rules are less restrictive. Many people attending the meeting viewed the proposed code revisions as just another way the government tries to control the people, and predicted that the proposal was a way for the City to identify food producers and tax them.

Additional angry opposition to the proposed code amendments came from other local food producers in reaction to the low number of animals permitted in the draft amendments. These numbers had been significantly reduced by City staff in response to the objections of the three opposing neighborhood association presidents.

The local daily newspaper and television news covered the raucous community meetings and reported what people said without any regard to the accuracy of their comments (DaRonco 2014a). A blogger for the daily newspaper created a very informative info-graphic that explained the amendments well (Billings 2014), which was distributed in the "lifestyle" section in a Sunday edition, but the news stories were quite inaccurate overall, reporting on the opinions of frustrated meeting attendees without inclusion of background or reference to the actual text of the proposed amendments.

The final community meeting in October, 2014 was lightly attended; the media did not cover the event. The City's zoning staff reported that as a result of the outcry at the previous meetings, the Urban Animal Unit approach would be reinstated, and that this would be reflected in a final draft that staff would present to the Planning Commission in early 2015. However, in early 2015 other zoning issues took precedence; a new draft was not released until May 2015, with Planning Commission public hearings scheduled for August. At this writing, the hearing is a few weeks away. The Planning Commission hearing will be followed by additional revision if necessary and consideration by Mayor and Council, anticipated in late 2015.

A Framework for Understanding the Culture of Policy Making

As policy is an important component of the ecology of obesity, understanding the policy making process is key to planning and executing efforts to address obesity. The process of policy making goes far beyond knowing the legal procedures for creating laws. Policymaking is a social and cultural endeavor and like any other social or cultural endeavor, demands competence from participants if they wish to succeed.

The Policy Team utilized the Multiple Streams theoretical framework of the policy process to guide its work. This framework was derived from the work of John Kingdon (2003) and outlined in Eisenberg (2011). Briefly, the framework posits policy making as a social and cultural endeavor that involves "three streams" of situations and actors that must converge in order to bring about policy change. The "problem stream" is closest to the lived experience of the issue being considered, and includes the people most impacted by the policy being considered as well as researchers who study the issue at the community level. The main contribution of problem stream players is voicing of a problem that needs to be solved. The "policy stream" consists of policy experts who know the issue—government staff, advocacy groups and coalitions, and lobbyists. Their main contribution is proposing alternative policy solutions. Finally, the "political" stream includes the officials who have the power to enact policy change and the political climate in which they operate. The final policy decision is made in the political stream; their main concern is balancing the interests of community constituencies and getting re-elected (Eisenberg 2011, 103–106).

The Policy Team used this framework to develop its work plan. In accordance with the Multiple Streams Framework, the "problem stream" was conceptualized as the people who support urban agriculture and whose activities would be impacted by policy change, as well as their neighbors. The "policy stream" was conceptualized as the people engaged in identifying alternative policy responses, primarily the City staff responsible for developing the zoning code amendments and any other individuals or entities they consult with, including the Planning Commission, Clarion Associates, and outspoken advocates from local organizations interested in food, sustainability, and environmental issues. The "political stream" was identified as the Mayor and City Council members and their staff. Throughout the project the Policy Team strived to understand how social actors in each stream conceptualized the urban agriculture zoning issue and provided information to inform their opinions and address their concerns. The Policy Team leader viewed her role as being a "social network integrator," connecting the players and ideas that originated within each of the three streams and facilitating communication among the streams, thus promoting convergence and policy action.

Issues in the Problem Stream

Problem stream concerns center around the impact a policy has on everyday life. The zoning code revision effort was initiated in the problem stream. Other CPPW teams working at the grassroots in targeted neighborhoods to develop urban food production activities provided the impetus for identifying the policy barriers to urban agriculture, which brought zoning issues to the forefront of the Policy Team's agenda. The CPPW Teams were also essential in connecting the Policy Team to the lived experience at the grassroots, which enabled us to document current practices that were occurring outside of the existing rules. CLUCKS was developed to support communication among animal keepers, as a tool for collecting stories and opinions about current practice, and as a conduit to provide grassroots stakeholders with information about the policy.

A shortcoming of the Policy Team's approach in the problem stream was that the initial conceptualization of the problem came from the perspective of individuals identified by the Neighborhood and Food Systems teams, and not from a broader representation of urban food producers. One segment of the food-producing constituency that was overlooked was food producers who subscribe to libertarian ideals and are not prone to joining organizations or Facebook groups, or participating in community projects. This group highly values self-sufficiency and so is deeply engaged in personal food production, but they are not part of the loose network of local food producers and advocates that operates around the local Food Bank. They had not been touched by efforts to educate the public about existing zoning rules that restrict what property owners can do and were mistakenly under the impression that the proposed rules would deprive them of their rights. Participation by many of these individuals in the community meetings was strong, boisterous, angry, and unexpected.

Issues in the Policy Stream

Policy stream concerns center on identifying alternative solutions and finding consensus for an approach. The Policy Team strived to become recognized by City zoning staff as a trusted source of information and alternative solutions. By providing high quality information in a format that was useful to City staff, the Policy Team did have a significant voice in identifying alternative policy approaches. However, it was remiss in not paying more attention to the neighborhood associations as actors in the policy stream. Rather, these organizations were assumed to be part of the problem stream. Presentations and meetings had been conducted with some associations and the project had been well received, but the system of neighborhood associations, the interaction among associations, and nuances of how particular associations interact with the City had not been addressed—with disastrous results. A more complete understanding of the influential policy stream actors in Tucson might have prompted the Policy Team to identify opposing neighborhood association presidents earlier and take steps to diffuse their concerns. This misstep set the policy-changing process back a full year, and is an example of the importance of cultural competence in how applied social scientists approach policy change. Had we done a better job of conceptualizing the problem and policy streams at the outset, much time could have been saved. The silver lining of the year-long delay was that it culminated in the public meetings that, while contentious, clearly demonstrated broad support for more, not less agricultural activity at the neighborhood level.

Issues in the Political Stream

While the problem stream was the impetus for Policy Team involvement, the City staff became engaged in urban agriculture at the behest of the political stream. Mayor and Council had instructed them to embark on the Sustainable Zoning Code project in early 2010, although food production was low priority within that project until the Policy Team presented staff with the draft Fact Sheets. Additionally, the City had been required to update its 10-year land use plan, which generated a separate set of community meetings from March 2011 through June 2013. The Policy Team was active in the "Plan Tucson" process as well, and facilitated the participation of many urban food producers. As a result, Plan Tucson (City of Tucson 2013) included a section on urban agriculture that called on the City to remove policy barriers in the zoning code. Tucson voters approved Plan Tucson in November 2013, thus creating a strong political stream rationale for pursuing the zoning code amendments.

Relationships between the Policy Team and the political stream actors had been nurtured well before this project was developed. The Team leader had been active (though not a central player) in political campaigns and the local Democratic party for many years, and was known to some, but not all of the political stream actors prior to scheduling formal informational meetings about the zoning code issues. This was an important factor that enhanced the ability of the Team to communicate with key policymakers. For example, involvement in the political stream provided opportunities for informal conversations about the zoning amendments during social and political events.

Although Mayor and Council generally supported an expansion of urban agricultural activity within city limits, from the beginning their enthusiasm was tempered by their expectations that certain neighborhood associations would strongly object, particularly to the animal rules. The local level political actors were far more informed about the policy and political streams landscape than the Policy Team had been.

When media reports of the controversial public meetings surfaced, some councilmembers withdrew support for any zoning code changes (DaRonco 2014b). Even though they had been individually briefed on how the new Code removes barriers to animal keeping that are in the current code, their response to the community outcry was to support the status quo—to abandon efforts to revise the Code. Their response was predictably political, demonstrating more concern with voter support than with the facts. The Mayor and other councilmembers agreed to withhold judgment until the completion of the process. The Mayor referred to the zoning code amendment process as "the great chicken debacle" in a conversation with this author in the fall of 2014.

LESSONS LEARNED

From an anthropological perspective, Shore and Wright (1997, 7) observe that policies "encapsulate the entire history and culture of the society that generated them." Clearly this is true for the policies that created an obesogenic environment in American cities. Current day obesity issues in Tucson, Arizona can be traced to public health issues that arose in other cities in the late nineteenth century and led to land use policy interventions, adopted nation-wide, that pushed agricultural uses into rural areas. When coupled with food industry developments, changes in transportation policy and systems, the westward expansion into areas where cheap land was available, and economic and social policy that puts some segments of the population at risk, Tucson developed to be a city characterized by urban sprawl, food deserts, and increasingly growing waistlines.

Changing current day zoning rules is a social and cultural endeavor that requires competency in all three streams engaged in the policy process. Anthropologists, who typically work within the problem stream, have long debated their role in policy development. While social science research often reveals and informs issues in the problem stream at the daily context, systems, and policy levels of the ecological model that deserve attention, the degree to which social scientists play a role in developing new policy and systems is a matter of personal choice and opportunity. A continuum of engagement in the policy process for social scientists (Eisenberg 2011, 111) ranges from simply distributing research findings among problem stream actors, to running for public office.

For social scientists that are committed to robust engagement in the policy process, the successes and failures of the efforts described above demonstrate that local level policy change is indeed possible, but requires a long-term commitment to both the community and to the project. It requires "showing up" in all three streams, providing high quality information in formats that are meaningful to the actors in all three streams, being perceived as a trusted actor in each stream, and being willing to make a long-term time commitment to the issue.

While the Tucson Sustainable Zoning Code amendments for urban agriculture have yet to be approved, the involvement of the Policy team over the past four years did create significant changes in the policy environment for urban agriculture. Urban agriculture is now squarely on the policy agenda. Enforcement of prohibitive zoning rules has eased at the County and City levels, and new, more permissive interpretations of the existing zoning code based on the ethnographic information about animal keeping have been adopted. Policy stream players have been educated about food access, food production, and the value of home- and community-level food production. Additionally, many problem stream food producers have learned about and participated in the policy process who had never done so before.

Of course, amending the Tucson zoning code to remove barriers to neighborhood food production and distribution will not, in itself, reverse the obesity epidemic in Tucson. Intervention at all levels of the ecological model of obesity will be necessary to make meaningful progress toward a community that supports a healthy lifestyle. Among the many activities undertaken as a result of the CPPW project were increasing the number of farmers' markets, providing food production training to more than 3500 people in high risk neighborhoods, establishing a system that provides healthy snacks to childcare providers, placing "produce bars" in 59 school lunch rooms, integrating physical activity to the school day, integrating nutrition education into the general curriculum, and providing playground and facility enhancements that encourage healthy physical activity in schools. Wellness programs were established in 379 worksites, reaching over 88,000 employees, and in 183 faith-based organizations reaching 108,000 parishioners. The activities of Pima County's CPPW grant, predicated on an ecological model of body weight, laid the groundwork for community action on policy and systems that continues three years after the grant ended and in the long-term will change the ecology of body weight, making it easier for people to choose a healthy lifestyle in generations to come.

References

Adams, Elizabeth J., Laurence Grummer-Strawn, and Gilberto Chavez. 2003. "Food Insecurity is Associated with Increased Risk of Obesity in California Women." *The Journal of Nutrition* 133(4): 1070–74.

Agne, April A., Rebecca Daubert, Maria L. Munoz, Isabel Scarinci, and Andrea L. Cherrington. 2012. "The Cultural Context of Obesity: Exploring Perceptions of Obesity and Weight Loss Among Latina Immigrants." *Journal of Immigrant & Minority Health* 14(6): 1063–70.

Al-Goblan, Abdullah S., Mohammed A. Al-Alfi, and Muhammad Z. Khan. 2014. "'Mechanism Linking Diabetes Mellitus and Obesity." *Diabetes Metabolic Syndrome and Obesity* 7: 587–91.

Allen, Bill. 2012. "Covering Nature and Society in Costa Rica." *Covering Nature and Society in Costa Rica.* Accessed July 24, 2013. http://mucostarica.wordpress.com/2012/01/02/monteverde-study-linksecotourism-to-reduced-food-security/.

Allison, D. B., V. C. Basile, and H. E. Yuker. 1991. "The Measurement of Attitudes toward and Beliefs about Obese Persons." *International Journal of Eating Disorders* 10(5): 599–607.

American Anthropological Association (AAA). 2015. Anthrosource. Accessed August 27, 2015. http://www.aaanet.org/publications/anthrosource/.

American Public Health Association. 2014. "Policy Database." Accessed December 31, 2014. http://www.apha.org/policies-and-advocacy/public-health-policy-statements/policy-database.

American Society for Metabolic and Bariatric Surgery (ASMBS). 2013. *New Evidence Prompts Update to Metabolic and Bariatric Surgery Clinical Guidelines.* Accessed August 27, 2015. http://asmbs.org/2013/04/new-evidence-prompts-update-to-metabolic-and-bariatric-surgery-clinical-guidelines/.

American Society for Metabolic and Bariatric Surgery (ASMBS). 2014. *Estimate of Bariatric Surgery Numbers.* Accessed August 27, 2015. https://asmbs.org/resources/estimate-of-bariatric-surgery-numbers.

An, Ruopeng. 2014. "Prevalence and Trends of Adult Obesity in the US, 1999–2012." *ISRN Obesity* 185132. doi:10.1155/2014/185132.

Andrade, Marta Cleia, and Daniela Cristina Alves. 2013. "Cooperativismo e Agricultura Familiar: Um Estudo de Caso." *Revista de Administração IMED* 3(3): 194–208.

Andreyeva, T., R. Sturm, and J.S. Ringel. 2004. "Moderate and Severe Obesity Have Large Differences in Health Care Costs." *Obesity Research* 12(12): 1936–43.

Apovian, Caroline M. 2013. "The Clinical and Economic Consequences of Obesity." *American Journal of Managed Care.* 19(11 Suppl): s219–28.

Armelagos, George. 2010. "The Omnivore's' Dilemma: The Evolution of the Brain and the Determinants of Food Choice." *Journal of Anthropological Research* 66(2): 161–86.

Armstrong, D. L. 2000. "A Community Diabetes Education and Gardening Project to Improve Diabetes Care in a Northwest American Indian Tribe." *Diabetes Educator* 26(113): 113–120.

Atkins, D. (ed.) 1998. *Looking Queer: Body Image and Identity in Lesbian, Bisexual, Gay and Transgender Communities*. Binghamton, NY: Haworth.

Bahr Bugge, A. 2011. "Lovin' It? A Study of Youth and the Culture of Fast Food." *Food, Culture & Society* 14(1): 71–89.

Baldridge, D. 2001. "The Elder Indian Population and Long-Term Care." In *Promises to Keep: Public Health Policy for American Indians and Alaska natives in the 21st Century* edited by M.a.R. Dixon. Washington, DC:American Public Health Association.

Bandura, Albert. 2004. "Health Promotion by Social Cognitive Means." *Health Education and Behavior* 31(2): 143–64.

Baron, R. B. 2011. "Telling Patients they are Overweight or Obese: An Insult or an Effective Intervention?" *Archives of Internal Medicine* 171(4): 321–22.

Batsis, J. A., M. M. Clark, K. Grothe, F. Lopez-Jimenez, M. L. Collazo-Clavell, V. K. Somers, and M. G. Sarr. 2009. "Self-Efficacy after Bariatric Surgery for Obesity. A Population-based Cohort Study." *Appetite* 52(3): 637–45.

Batsis, J. A., F. Lopez-Jimenez, M. L. Collazo-Clavell, M. M. Clark, V. K. Somers, and M. G. Sarr. 2009. "Quality of Life after Bariatric Surgery: A Population-based Cohort Study." *American Journal of Medicine* 122(11): 1055.e1–1055.e10.

Batsis, J. A., A. Romero-Corral, M. L. Collazo-Clavell, M. G. Sarr, V. K. Somers, and F. Lopez-Jimenez. 2008. "Effect of Bariatric Surgery on the Metabolic Syndrome: A Population-Based, Long-Term Controlled Study." *Mayo Clinic Proceedings* 83(8): 897–906.

Batsis, J. A., M. G. Sarr, M. L. Collazo-Clavell, R. J. Thomas, A. Romero-Corral, V. K. Somers, and F. Lopez-Jimenez. 2008. "Cardiovascular Risk after Bariatric Surgery for Obesity." *American Journal of Cardiology* 102(7): 930–37.

Becker, A. E. 1995. *Body, Self, and Society: The View from Fiji*. Philadelphia: University of Pennsylvania Press.

Belle, S. H., W. Chapman, A. P. Courcoulas A. P., D. R. Flum, M. Gagner, W. B. Inabnet, W. C. King, J. E. Mitchell, E. J. Patterson, R. Thirlby, B. M. Wolfe, and S. Z. Yanovski. 2008. "Relationship of Body Mass Index with Demogrpahic and Clinical Characteristics in the Longitudinal Assessment of Bariatric Surgery (LABS)." *Surgery for Obesity and Related Diseases* 4(4): 474–80.

Benson, Peter. 2012. "Commentary: Biopolitical Injustice and Contemporary Capitalism." *American Ethnologist* 39(3): 488–90.

Benson, Peter. 2014. "Corporate Paternalism and the Problem of Harmful Products." *PoLAR: Political and Legal Anthropology Review* 37(2): 218–30.

Bent-Martin Eliassen, Marita Melhus, Ketil Lenert Hansen, Ann Ragnhild Broderstad. 2013. "Marginalisation and Cardiovascular Disease among Rural Sami in Northern Norway: a Population-Based Cross-Sectional Study." *BMC Public Health* 13(522): 9.

Bernard, Russell H. 2011. *Research Methods in Anthropology: Qualitative and Quantitative Approaches.* Lanham, MD: Altamira Press.

Better Business Bureau. 2014. "Children's Food & Beverage Advertising Initiative." Accessed June 25, 2015. https://www.bbb.org/globalassets/local-bbbs/council-113/media/cfbai/audience-definitions-aug-2014.pdf

Billings, Susan. 2014. "Urban Agriculture, A Closer Look at City's Proposals." *Arizona Daily Star,* June 30, 2014.

Birch, Eugene and Christopher Silver. 2009. "One Hundred Years of City Planning's Enduring and Evolving Connections." *Journal of the American Planning Association* 75(2): 113–22. doi: 10.1080/01944360902777031.

Bleich, S. N., K. A. Gudzune, W. L. Bennett, M. P. Jarlenski, and L. A. Cooper. 2013. "How Does Physician BMI Impact Patient Trust and Perceived Stigma?" *Preventative Medicine* 57(2): 120–24.

Blom-Hoffman, Jessica, Kaila R. Wilcox, Laim Dunn, Stephen S. Lee and Thomas Power. 2008. "Family Involvement in School-Based Health Promotion: Bringing Nutritional Information Home." *School Psychology Review* 37(4): 567–77.

Bocchieri, L. E., M. Meana, and B. L. Fisher. 2002. "Perceived Psychosocial outcomes of gastric bypass surgery: A qualitative study. *Obesity Surgery* 12(6): 781–88.

Boero, Natalie. 2010. "Bypassing Blame: Bariatric Surgery and the Case of Biomedical Failure." In *Biomedicalization: Technoscience, Health and Illness in the U.S.* A. E. Clarke, L. Mamo, J. R. Fosket, J. R. Fishman, and J. K. Shim, eds. Durham, NC: Duke University Press.

Boero, Natalie. 2012. *Killer Fat: Media, Medicine, and Morals in the American "Obesity Epidemic."* New Brunswick, NJ: Rutgers University Press.

Bombak, A. 2014. "Obesity, Health at Every Size, and Public Health Policy." *American Journal of Public Health* 104(2): e60–e67.

Bonell, Chris, Martin McKee, Adam Fletcher, Paul Wilkinson, and Andy Haines. 2011. "One Nudge Forward, Two Steps Back." *British Medical Journal* 342: d401.

Bordo, S. 1993. *Unbearable Weight: Feminism, Western Culture, and the Body.* Oakland, CA: University of California Press.

Borovoy, Amy, and Christina Roberto. 2015. "Japanese and American Public Health Approaches to Preventing Population Weight Gain: A Role for Paternalism?" *Social Science & Medicine* Accessed August 21, 2015. doi:10.1016/j.socscimed.2015.08.018.

Boumtje, Pierre I., Chung L. Huang, Jonq-Ying Lee, and Biing-Hwan Lin, 2005. "Dietary Habits, Demographics, and the Development of Overweight and Obesity among Children in the United States." *Food Policy* 30: 115–28. doi:10.1016/j.foodpol.2004.02.004

Bourdieu, Pierre. 1984. *Distinction: A Social Critique of the Judgement of Taste*. R. Nice, trans. Cambridge, MA: Harvard University Press.

Bourdieu, Pierre. 1986. "The Forms of Capital." In *Handbook of Theory and Research for the Sociology of Education*. J. Richardson, ed. Santa Barbara, CA: Greenwood.

Bowman, Shanty, Steven Gortmaker, Cara Ebbeling, Mark Pereira, and David Ludwig. 2004. "Effects of Fast-Food Consumption on Energy Intake and Diet Quality Among Children in a National Household Survey." *Pediatrics* 113(1): 112–19.

Boyle, J. P. 2010. "Projection of the Year 2050 Burden of Diabetes in the US Adult Population: Dynamic Modeling of Incidence, Mortality, and Prediabetes Prevalence." *Population Health Metrics* 8(29).

Brainard, Lael, ed. 2009. *Brazil is an Economic Superpower: Understanding Brazil's Role in the Global Economy*. Washington, DC: Brookings Institute Press.

Bray, George, Samara Nielsen, and Barry Popkin. 2003. "Consumption of high-fructose corn syrup in beverages may play a role in the epidemic of obesity." *American Journal of Clinical Nutrition* 79: 537–43.

Braziel, J. E. and K. Lebesco (eds). 2001. *Bodies Out of Bounds*. Santa Barbara, CA: University of California Press.

Brenton, Barrett. 2013. "In Focus: Biocultural Paradox of Hunger and Obesity: Implications for Food Security and Public Health Policy." *Anthropology News* 54(12): e8–e22.

Brewis, Alexandra. 1999. "Accuracy of Attractive Body Judgment." *Current Anthropology* 40: 548–53.

Brewis, Alexandra. 2003. "Biocultural Aspects of Obesity in Young Mexican Schoolchildren." *American Journal of Human Biology* 15(3): 446–60.

Brewis, Alexandra. 2011. *Obesity: Cultural and Biocultural Perspectives*. New Jersey: Rutgers University Press.

Brewis, Alexandra. 2012. "Obesity and Human Biology: Toward a Global Perspective." *American Journal of Human Biology* 24(3): 258–60.

Brewis, Alexandra. 2014. "Stigma as a Social Driver of Obesity." *Social Science and Medicine* 118: 152–158.

Brewis, Alexandra and S. T. McGarvey. 2000. "Body Image, Body Size, and Samoan Ecological and Individual Modernization." *Ecology of Food and Nutrition* 39(2): 105–20.

Brewis, Alexandra. and M. Gartin. 2006. "Biocultural Constructions of Obesogenic Ecologies of Childhood: Parental Feeding versus Young Child Eating Strategies." *American Journal of Human Biology* 18: 203–13.

Brewis, Alexandra and S. Lee. 2010. "Children's Work, Earnings, and Nutrition in Urban Mexican Shantytowns." *American Journal of Human Biology* 22(1): 60–68.

Brewis, Alexandra and Amber Wutich. 2014. "A World of Suffering? Biocultural Approaches too Fat Stigma in the Global Contexts of the Obesity Epidemic". Annals of Anthropological Practice 38: 269–83.

Brewis, Alexandra and Amber Wutich. 2012. "Implicit versus Explicit Fat-Stigma." *American Journal of Human Biology* 24: 332–38.

Brewis, Alexandra, Daniel Hruschka, and Amber Wutich. 2011. "Vulnerability to Fat-Stigma in Women's Everyday Relationships." *Social Science and Medicine* 73: 491–97.

Brewis, Alexandra, S. T. McGarvey, J. Jones, and B. Swinburn. 1997. "Perceptions of body size in Pacific Islanders." *International Journal of Obesity* 22: 185–89.

Brewis, Alexandra, Amber Wutich, Ashlan Falletta-Cowden, and Isa Rodriguez-Soto. 2011. "Body Norms and Fat Stigma in Global Perspective." *Current Anthropology* 52(2): 269–76.

Breyer, Betsy, and Adriana Voss-Andreae. 2013. "Food Mirages: Geographic and Economic Barriers to Healthful Food Access in Portland, Oregon." *Health and Place* 24(November): 131–39.

Brown, Peter J. 1991. "Culture and the Evolution of Obesity." *Human Nature* 2(1): 31–57.

Brownstein, J. N. 2007. "Effectiveness of Community Health Workers in the Care of People with Hypertension." *American Journal of Preventative Medicine* 32(5): 435–47.

Bronfenbrenner, Urie. 1977. "Toward an Experimental Ecology of Human Development." *American Psychologist* 32: 513–31.

Brooker, M. 2000. "Anthropological Aspects of Changing Beliefs Among the Obese." *Practicing Anthropology* 22(2): 8–12.

Brown, D. E., S. E. Hampson, J. P Dubanoski, A. S. Murai, and T. A. Hillier. 2009. "Effects of Ethnicity and Socioeconomic Status on Body Composition in an Admixed, Multiethnic Population in Hawaii." *American Journal of Human Biology* 21(3): 383–88.

Brown, Racine M. 2013. "'They Come, but They Don't Spend as Much Money': Livelihoods, Dietary Diversity, Food Security, and Nutritional Status in Two Roatan Communities in the Wake of Global Crises in Food Prices and Finance." PhD diss., University of South Florida.

Brownell, Kelly D., Rogan Kersh, David S. Ludwig, Robert C Post, Rebecca M. Puhl, Marlene B. Schwartz, and Walter C. Willett. 2010. "Personal Responsibility and Obesity: A Constructive Approach to a Controversial Issue." *Health Affairs* 29(3): 379–87.

Brownlee, Shannon. 2007. *Overtreated: Why Too Much Medicine is Making us Sicker and Poorer*. New York: Bloomsbury.

Brumberg, J. 1988. *Fasting Girls: the Emergence of Anorexia Nervosa as a Modern Disease*. Cambridge, MA: Harvard University Press.

Brune, J. A. and D. J. Wilson. 2013. *Disability and Passing: Blurring the Lines of Identity*. Philadelphia: Temple University Press.

Bryant, Carol A., Anita H. Courtney, Robert J. McDermott, Moya L. Alfonso, Julie A. Baldwin, Jen Nickleson, Kelli McCormack-Brown, Rita D. DeBate, Leah M. Phillips, Zachary Thompson, and Yiliang Zhu. 2009. " Promoting Physical Activity Among Youth Through Community Based-Prevention Marketing." *Journal of School Health* 80(5): 214–24.

Buchwald, H., Y. Avidor, E. Braunwald, M.D. Jensen, W. Pories, K. Fahrbach, and K. Schoelles. 2004. "Bariatric Surgery: A Systematic Review and Meta-Analysis." *Journal of the American Medical Association* 292(14): 1724–28.

Burdette, Hillary, Thomas Wadden, and Robert Whitaker. 2006. "Neighborhood Safety, Collective Efficacy, and Obesity in Women with Young Children." *Obesity* 14(3): 518–25.

Burgmer, R., T. Legenbauer, A. Muller, M. de Zwaan, C. Fischer, and S. Herpertz. 2014. "Psychological Outcomes 4 Years after Restrictive Bariatric Surgery." *Obesity Surgery* 2014 Mar 30. [Epub ahead of print.]

Burkhalter, Toni M., and Charles H. Hillman. 2011. "A Narrative Review of Physical Activity, Nutrition, and Obesity to Cognition and Scholastic Performance across the Human Lifespan." *Advances in Nutrition* 2(Suppl): 201S–206S.

Butterfoss, Frances D., and Michelle C. Kegler. 2009. "The Community Coalition Action Theory." In *Emerging Theories in Health Promotion Practice and Research: Strategies for Improving Public Health*, 2nd ed, edited by Ralph J. diClemente, Richard C. Crosby and Michelle C. Kegler, 237–76. San Francisco: Jossey-Bass.

Butto, Andrea, Isolda Dantas and Karla Hora. 2012. *As Mulhere nas Estatísticas Agripecuárias: Experiências nas países do Sul.* Brasília: Ministério de Desenvolvimento Agrário.

Câmara Interministerial de Segurança Alimentar e Nutricional (CAISAN). 2011. *Plano Nacional de Segurança Alimentar e Nutricional – 2012–2015* (Brasília: CAISIN).

Câmara Interministerial de Segurança Alimentar e Nutricional (CAISAN). 2014. *Estratégia Intersetorial de Prevenção e Controle de Obesidade: Recomendações para Estados e Municípios* (Brasília: CAISIN).

Campbell, John and Naoki Ikegami. 1998. *The Art of Balance in Health Policy.* Ann Arbor: University of Michigan Press.

Campbell, John Creighton, Naoki Ikegami, and Yusuke Tsugawa. 2014. "The Political-Historical Context of Japanese Health Care." In *Universal Health Coverage for Inclusive and Sustainable Development: Lessons from Japan*, edited by Naoki Ikegami, 1–13. Washington, D.C.: The World Bank.

Campbell, Ruth, 1996. "The Three-Minute Cure: Doctors and Elderly Patients in Japan." In *Containing Health Care Costs in Japan,* edited by Naoki Ikegami and John Creighton Campbell, 226–33. Ann Arbor: University of Michigan Press.

Campos, P. 2004. *The Obesity Myth: Why America's Obsession with Weight is Hazardous to Your Health.* London: Penguin Group.

Cantor, Allison, Jenny Pena, and David Himmelgreen. 2013. "'We Never Ate Like That, Not Fast Food, or Junk Foods': Accounts of Changing Maternal Diet in a Tourist Community in Rural Costa Rica." *Ecology of Food And Nutrition* 52(6): 479–96.

Carney, Patricia A., Janet L. Hamada, Rebecca Rdesinski, Lorena Sprager, Katelyn R. Nichols, Betty Y. Liu, Joel Pelayo, Maria Antonia Sanchez, and Jacklien Shannon. 2012. "Impact of a Community Gardening Project on Vegetable Intake, Food Security and Family Relationships: a Community-Based Participatory Research Study." *Journal of Community Health* 37(4): 874–81.

Carpenter, K. M., D. S. Hasin, D. B. Allison, and M. S. Faith. 2000. "Relationships between Obesity and DSM-IV Major Depressive Disorder, Suicide Ideation, and

Suicide Attempts: Results from a general population study." *American Journal of Public Health* 90: 251–57.

Carrel, A. 2005. "Effects of Nutrition Education and Exercise in Obese Children: the Ho-Chunk Youth Fitness Program." *World Medical Journal* 104(5): 44–47.

Carryer, J. 1997. "A Feminist Appraisal of the Experience of Embodied Largeness: A Challenge for Nursing." Doctoral Dissertation, Massey University.

Casper, M. J. and L. J. Moore. 2009. *Missing Bodies: The Politics of Visibility*. New York: New York University Press.

Cassels, Susan. 2006. "Overweight in the Pacific: Links Between Foreign Dependence, Global Food Trade, and Obesity in the Federated States of Micronesia." *Globalization and Health* 2: 10.

Catalani, Caricia, and Meredith Minkler. 2009. "Photovoice: A Review of the Literature in Health and Public Health." *Health Education & Behavior*. doi: 10.1177/1090198109342084.

Centers for Disease Control and Prevention. 2007. *Take Charge of Your Diabetes*, 4th ed., Atlanta: U.S. Department of Health and Human Services, 2007.

Centers for Disease Control and Prevention. 2014. "Childhood Obesity Facts." Prevalence of Childhood Obesity in the United States, 2011–2012. Accessed August 7, 2014. Available from http://www.cdc.gov/obesity/data/childhood.html.

Centers for Disease Control and Prevention, 2014a. "Obesity and Overweight, Causes and Consequences." Accessed December 30, 2014. http://www.cdc.gov/obesity/adult/causes/index.html

Centers for Disease Control and Prevention. 2014b. "Physical Activity, How Much Physical Activity Do Adults Need?" Accessed December 20, 2014. http://www.cdc.gov/physicalactivity/everyone/guidelines/adults.html

Centers for Disease Control and Prevention, Division of Community Health. 2014c. "Making Healthy Living Easier." Accessed December 20, 2014. http://www.cdc.gov/nccdphp/dch/index.htm

Chaddad, Fabio R., and Marcos S. Jank. 2006. "The Evolution of Agricultural Policies and Agribusiness Development in Brazil." *Choices* 21(2): 85–90.

Chandon, Pierre, and Brian Wansink. 2010. "Is Food Marketing Making Us Fat? A Multi-Disciplinary Review." *Foundations and Trends in Marketing* 5(3): 113–96. doi: 10.1561/1700000016

Cherneff, Jill B. R., and Eve Hochwald. 2006. *Visionary Observers: Anthropological Inquiry and Education*, Lincoln, NE: University of Nebraska Press.

Cherry, Colleen O'Brien, Elizabeth Serieux, Martin Didier, Mary Elizabeth Nuttal, and Richard J. Schuster. 2014. "Prevalence of Risk Factors for the Metabolic Syndrome in the Middle Income Caribbean Nation of St. Lucia." *Advances in Preventive Medicine* 2014: 5. doi: 10.1155/2014/501972.

Chollett, D. L. 2014. "The Native American Organic Garden: Using Service Learning as a Site of Resistance." *Culture, Agriculture, Food and Environment* 36(2): 93–104.

Christakis, Nicholas A., and James H. Fowler. 2007. "The Spread of Obesity in a Large Social Network Over 32 Years." *New England Journal of Medicine* 357: 370–79.

Christensen, B. J. 2012. "Problem Solving or Problem Bypass? A qualitative interview study assessing treatment results after gastric bypass surgery." *The Complexity of Obesity Proceedings: International Conference on Obesity and Quality of Life Outcomes.* 5–7 June 2012. Balestrand: Norway.

Christeson, William, Amy Taggert, Soren Messner-Zidell, Mike Kiernan, Judy Kusick, and Ryan Day. 2012. "Mission Readiness: Still Too Fat To Fight." Council for a Strong America. Accessed December 30, 2014. http://www.rwjf.org/content/dam/farm/reports/reports/2012/rwjf401381.

Christopher, A. N., R. D. Morgan, P. Marek, J. D. Troisi, J. R. Jones, and D. F. Reinhart. 2005. "Affluence Cues and First Impressions: Does it Matter How the Affluence was Acquired?" *Journal of Economic Psychology* 26(2): 187–200.

City of São Paulo. Plano Director. Accessed August 27, 2015. http://www.prefeitura.sp.gov.br/cidade/secretarias/desenvolvimento_urbano/legislacao/plano_diretor/index.php.

City of São Paulo. Regularização das Feiras Livres Complete 100 Anos na Cidade. Accessed June 12, 2015. http://www.capital.sp.gov.br/portal/noticia/3599#ad-image-0.

City of Tucson. 2013. "Indicators of Neighborhood Stress." Accessed December 30, 2014. http://hcd.tucsonaz.gov/hcd/indicators-neighborhood-stress.

City of Tucson. "Plan Tucson, City of Tucson General and Sustainability Plan." Accessed January 3, 2015. http://oip.tucsonaz.gov/files/integrated-planning/Plan_Tucson_Complete_Doc_11-13-13.pdf.

City of Tucson. 1995. "Land Use Code". City of Tucson Code: Chapter 23. Accessed January 3, 2015. https://www.tucsonaz.gov/files/pdsd/codes-ordinances/Complete_LUC_Sept2012.pdf.

Clark, C. M., Jr. 2001. "The National Diabetes Education Program, Changing the Way Diabetes is Treated: Comprehensive Diabetes Care." *Diabetes Care* 24(4): 617–18.

Clínica Naturista de Medicina Integral. "Nutrición: Alimentación Saludable (Nutrition: Healthy Eating)" Accessed January 10, 2015. http://www.youtube.com/watch?v=GU8WFy9io4Y&feature=youtu.be.

Cohen, A. P. (ed). 1994. *Signifying Identities: Anthropological perspectives on boundaries and contested values*. London: Routledge.

Colditz, G. A. 1992. "Economic costs of obesity." *The American Journal of Clinical Nutrition* 55(2suppl.): 503s.

Coleman Karen, Maggie Shordon, Susan Caparosa, Magdalena Pomichowski, and David Dzewaltowski. 2012. "The Health Options for Nutrition Environments in Schools (Healthy ONES) Group Randomized Trial: Using Implementation of Models of Change for Nutrition Policy and Environments in Low-Income Schools." *International Journal of Behavioral Nutrition and Physical Activity* 9: 80.

Collazo-Clavell, M. L. 2008. "Bariatric Surgery: important considerations for the primary care provider." *Comprehensive Therapy* 34(3–4): 159–65.

Collazo-Clavell, M. L., A. Jimenez, S. F. Hodgson, and M. G. Sarr. 2004. "Osteomalacia after Roux-en-Y Gastric Bypass." *Endocrine Practice* 10(3): 195–98.

Conde, Wonley L. and Carlos A. Monteiro. 2014. "Nutrition Transition and Double Burden of Undernutrition and Excess of Weight in Brazil." *The American Journal of Clinical Nutrition* 100(6): 1617S–22S.

Confederação Nacional da Indústria/Serviço Social da Indústria Departamento Nacional. 2008. *Programa SESI Cozinha Brasil: A Receita de Cidadania*. Brasília: SESI).

CONSEA. 2010. A *Segurança Alimentar e Nutricional e o Direto Humano à Alimentação Adequada no Brasil* (Brasília: Government of Brazil).

Conti, K. M. 2006. "Diabetes Prevention in Indian Country: Developing Nutrition Models to Tell the Story of Food-System Change." *Journal of Transcultural Nursing* 17(3): 234–45.

Cordain, Lauren, S. Boyd Eaton, Anthony Sebastian, Neil Mann, Staffan Lindeberg, Bruce A. Watkins, James H. O'Keefe, and Janette Brand-Miller. 2005. "Origins and Evolution of the Western Diet: Health Implications for the 21st Century." *American Journal of Clinical Nutrition* 81: 341–54.

Costello, Anthony, and Alimuddin Zumla. 2000. "Moving to Research Partnerships in Developing Countries." British Medical Journal 321: 827–29.

Council on Foreign Relations. 2014. "The Emerging Global Health Crisis." Council on Foreign Relations Press.

Courcoulas, A. P., N. J. Christian, S. H. Belle, P. D. Berk, D. R. Flum, L. Gracia, M. Horlick, M. A. Kalarchian, W. C. King, J. E. Mitchell, E. J. Patterson, J. R. Pender, A. Pomp, W. J. Pories, R. C. Thirlby, S. Z. Yanovski, and B. M. Wolfe. 2013. "Weight Change and Health Outcomes at 3 Years after Bariatric Surgery among Individuals with Severe Obesity." *Journal of the American Medical Association* 310(22): 2416–25.

Crespo, Noe C., John P. ELder, Guadalupe X. Ayala, Nadia R. Campbell, ELva M. Arredondo, Donald J. Slymen, Barbara Baquero, James F. Sallis, and Thomas L. McKenzie. 2012. "'Results of a Multi-level Intervention to Prevent and Control Childhood Obesity among Latino Children: The Aventuras Para Niños Study." *Annals of Behavioral Medicine* 43(1): 84–100.

Crooks, Deborah. 2003. "Trading Nutrition for Education: Nutritional Status and the Sale of Snack Foods in an Eastern Kentucky School." *Medical Anthropology Quarterly* 17(2): 182–99.

Crooks, Deborah. 2000. "Food Consumption, Activity, and Overweight among Elementary School Children in an Appalachian Kentucky Community." *American Journal of Physical Anthropology* 112(2): 159–70.

Dahl, B. 2014. "'Too Fat to be an Orphan': The Moral Semiotics of Food Aid in Botswana." *Cultural Anthropology* 29(4): 626–47.

Dantos, Isolda. 2005. "A Construção da Economia Feminista na Rede Xique-Xique."*Gerando Riquezas e Novos Valores. Revista Agriculturas* 2(3): 27–30.

Dapice, A. N. 2006. "The Medicine Wheel." *Journal of Transcultural Nursing* 17(3): 251–60.

DaRonco, Darren. 2014a. "Urban Farming Supporters Decry Proposed Amendments." *Arizona Daily Star,* June 11, 2014.

DaRonco, Darren. 2014b. "City May Ditch Proposed Rules on Agriculture." *Arizona Daily Star,* July 1, 2014.

Davidson, L.K. and D.M. Gitlitz. 2002. *Pilgrimage: From the Ganges to Graceland: An Encyclopedia, Volume 1*. ABC-CLIO.

Dawkins, M. A. 2012. *Clearly Invisible: Racial Passing and the Color of Cultural Identity*. Waco, TX: Baylor University Press.

Department of Health and Human Services. 2011. *National Diabetes Education Program: An Overview.*

Deutsch, Tracey. 2012. "Labor Histories of Food." In *The Oxford Handbook of Food History,* edited by Jeffrey Pilcher, 61–80. Oxford: Oxford University Press.

Diem, R. A., and J. E. Davis. 2013. *Sustainability, Growth, and Globalization: A Social Science Perspective.* Charlotte: Information Age Publishing, Inc.

Dietz, William H. 1995. "Does Hunger Cause Obesity?." *Pediatrics* 95(5): 766–67.

Dinour, Lauren M., Dara Bergen, and Ming-Chin Yeh. 2007. "The food insecurity–obesity paradox: a review of the literature and the role food stamps may play."*Journal of the American Dietetic Association* 107(11): 1952–61.

Drake, H. Max. 1989. "Using Stakeholders in the Research Process: A Case Study in Human Services." In *Making Our Research Useful: Case Studies in the Utilization of Anthropological Knowledge,* edited by John van Willigen, Barbara Rylko-Bauer, and Ann McElroy, 237–55. Boulder, CO: Westview.

Dressler, W. W., K. S. Oths, R. P. Ribeiro, M. C. Balieiro, and J. E. Dos Santos. 2008. "Cultural Consonance and Adult Body Composition in Urban Brazil." *American Journal of Human Biology* 20(1): 15–22.

Drewnowski, Adam. 2004. "Obesity and the Food Environment: Dietary Energy Density and Diet Costs." *American Journal of Preventive Medicine* 27(3S): 154–62.

Drewnowski, Adam. 2009. "Obesity, Diets, and Social Inequalities." *Nutrition Reviews* 67(suppl 1): S36–S39.

Drewnowski, Adam, Colin Rehm, and David Solet. 2009. "Disparities in Obesity Rates: Analysis by ZIP Code Area." *Social Science & Medicine* 65: 2458–63. doi:10.1016/j.socscimed.2007.07.001.

Duarte, Gisléia Benini, Berno Sampaio, and Yony Sampaio. 2009. "Programa Bolsa Família: Impacto das Transferências Sobre os Gastos com Alimentos em Famílias Rurais." *Revista de Economia e Sociologia Rural* 47(4): 903–18.

Duerler T., and G. Maskarinec. 2007. "Public Health in the Republic of Palau: What We Can Learn from a Small Island Country." *Pacific Health Dialog* 14(1): 182–87.

Durkin, A. J., M. Bloomston, M. M. Murr, and A. S. Rosemurgy. 1999. "Financial Status Does not Predict Weight Loss after Bariatric Surgery." *Obesity Surgery* 9(6): 524–26.

Dutton, G. R., Tan, F., Perri, M., Stine, C. C., Dancer-Brown, M., Goble, M. & Van Vessen, N. 2010. "What Words Should We Use When Discussing Excess Weight?" *Journal of the American Board of Family Medicine* 23(5): 606–13.

Earvolino-Ramirez, M. 2008. Living with Bariatric Surgery: Totally Different but Still Evolving. *Bariatric Nursing and Surgical Patient Care* 3(1): 17–25.

Edmonds, A. 2010. *Pretty Modern: Beauty, Sex, and Plastic Surgery in Brazil.* Durham, NC: Duke University Press.

Edwards, K. and B. Patchell. 2009. "State of the Science: a Cultural View of Native Americans and Diabetes Prevention." *Journal of Cultural Diversity* 16(1): 32–35.

Eisenberg, Merrill. 2011. "Medical Anthropology and Public Policy." In *A Companion to Medical Anthropology,* edited by Merrill Singer and Pamela Erickson, 93–116. Chichester: Wiley-Blackwell

Eisenberg, Merrill. 2014. "Zoning Into Urban Agriculture." *Edible Baja Arizona* 1(4): 42.

Elder, J. P. 2013. "Mexico and the USA: The World's Leaders in the Obesity Epidemic." *Salud Pública de México* 55(Suppl 3): 355.

Ellis, G. 2005. "St. Lucia's Declining Banana Trade." *BBC News*. Accessed August 27, 2015. http://news.bbc.co.uk/2/hi/americas/4737473.stm.

Engebretson, J., J. Mahoney and E. D. Carlson. 2008. "Cultural Competence in the Era of Evidence-Based Practice." *Journal of Professional Nursing* 24(3): 172–78.

Encinosa, W., D. Du, and D. Bernard. 2011. "Anti-Obesity Drugs and Bariatric Surgery." In *The Oxford Handbook of the Social Science of Obesity*. J. Cawley, editor. London: Oxford University Press.

Ennis, Sharon R., Mararys Rios-Vargas, and Nora G. Albert. 2011. "The Hispanic Population: 2010: 2010 Census Briefs." Accessed December 16, 2014. http://www.census.gov/prod/cen2010/briefs/c2010br-04.pdf.

Erikson, E. H. 1972. *Childhood and Society*. London: Penguin Books.

Estevez-Abe, Margarita, 2008. *Welfare and Capitalism in Postwar Japan*. Cambridge: Cambridge University Press.

Evenson, Kelly, Richard Block, Ana Roux, Aileen McGin, Fang Wen, and Daniel Rodriguez. 2012. "Associations of Adult Physical Activity with Perceived Safety and Police-recorded Crime: the Multi-ethnic Study of Atherosclerosis." *Journal of Behavioral Nutrition and Physical Activity* 9: 146–58. doi: 10.1186/1479-5868-9-146.

Everett, Margaret. 2011. "Practicing Anthropology on a Community-Based Public Health Coalition: Lessons from HEAL." *Annals of Anthropological Practice* 35(2): 10–26.

Everett, Margaret. and J. N. Wieland. 2012. "Diabetes among Oaxaca's Transnational Population: An Emerging Syndemic." *Annals of Anthropological Practice* 36(2): 295–311.

Fallon, A. 1990. "Culture in the Mirror: Sociocultural determinants of body image." In *Body Images: Development, Deviance, and Change*. T. F. Cash and T. Pruzinsky, eds. New York: Guilford.

FAO. 2014a. "Thirteen Countries Move Closer to Eradicating Hunger." Rome, November 30. Accessed January 2, 2015. http://www.fao.org/news/story/en/item/270380/icode/.

FAO. 2014b. "The State of Food Insecurity in the World." Rome. Accessed January 2, 2015. http://www.fao.org/3/a-i4030e.pdf.

Fardouly J. and L. R. Vartanian. 2012. "Changes in Weight Bias Following Weight Loss: the impact of weight-loss method." *International Journal of Obesity* 36(2): 314–19.

Farrell, A. E. 2011. *Fat Shame: Stigma and the Fat Body in American Culture*. New York: New York University Press.

Feather, N. T. and S. Dawson. 1998. "Judging Deservingness and Affect in Relation to Another's Employment or Unemployment: a test of a justice model." *European Journal of Social Psychology* 28(3): 361–81.

Fechner, Mary J. 2011. "Berliners' Models of Heart Disease Causation." *Qualitative Health Research* 21(6): 11. doi: 10.1177/1049732311400430.

Fee, H. R. and M. R. Nusbaumer. 2012. "Social Distance and the Formerly Obese: Does the Stigma of Obesity Linger?" *Sociological Inquiry* 82: 356–77.

Feighery E., and T. Rogers. 1990. "Building & Maintaining Effective Coalitions." Palo Alto: Stanford Health Promotion Research Center.

Feira do Ibirapuera. Accessed June 13, 2015. https://www.facebook.com/feira.ibirapuera/.

Feldman, Eric, 2001. "The Landscape of Japanese Tobacco Policy: Law, Smoking and Social Change." *The American Journal of Comparative Law* 49: 679–706.

Feng, Jing, Thomas Glass, Frank Curriero, Walter Stewart, and Brian Schwartz. 2010. "The Built Environment and Obesity: A Systematic Review of the Epidemiologic Evidence." *Health and Place* 16: 175–90. doi:10.1016/j.healthplace.2009.09.008.

Ferrira, M. L. and G. C. Lang, eds. 2006. *Indigenous Peples and Diabetes: Community Empowerment and Wellness*. Durhan, NC: Carolina Academic Press.

Ferzacca, S. 2012. "Diabetes and Culture." *Annual Review of Anthropology* 41: 411–426.

Ferzacca, S. 2000. "'Actually, I Don't Feel that Bad': Managing Diabetes and the Clinical Encounter." *Medical Anthropology Quarterly* 14(1): 28–50.

Finkelstein, Eric, Justin Trogdon, Joel W. Cohen, and William Dietz. 2009. "Annual Medical Spending Attributable To Obesity: Payer-And Service-Specific Estimates." *Health Affairs* 28(5): w822–31. doi: 10.1377/hlthaff.28.5.w822.

Fisher, Andy. 1999. "Hot Peppers and Parking Lot Peaches: Evaluating Farmers' Markets in Low Income Communities." Report of the Community Food Security Coalition, January 1999. Accessed August 24, 2015. http://www.eatbettermovemore.org/SA/enact/neighborhood/documents/community.farmersmarkets.tools.hotpepperspeaches.pdf.

Fitzgerald, N. 2010. "Acculturation, Socioeconomic Status, and Health among Hispanics." *Annals of Anthropological Practice* 34(1): 28–46.

Flegel, Katherine M., Margaret Carroll, Robert J. Kuczmarski, and Clifford L. Johnson. 1998. "Overweight and Obesity in the United States: Prevalence and Trends, 1960–1994." *International Journal of Obesity and Related Metabolic Disorders*, 22: 39–47.

Flegal, Katherine M., Margaret D. Carroll, Brian K. Kit, and Cynthia L. Ogden. 2012. "Prevalence of Obesity and Trends in the Distribution of Body Mass Index Among U.S. Adults, 1999–2010." *Journal of the American Medical Association* 307(5): 491–97.

Fleischhacker, S. E., K. R. Evenson, D. A. Rodriguez, and A. S. Ammerman. 2011. "A Systematic Review of Fast Food Access Studies." *Obesity Reviews* 12: e460–71. doi: 10.1111/j.1467-789X.2010.00715.x.

Flum, D. R., S. H. Belle, W. C. King, A. S. Wahed, P. Berk, W. Chapman, W. Pories, A. Courcoulas, C. McCloskey, J. Mitchell, E. Patterson, A. Pomp, M. A. Staten, S. Z. Yanovski, R. Thirlby, and B. Wolfe. 2009. Perioperative safety in the longitudinal assessment of bariatric surgery. *New England Journal of Medicine* 361(5): 445–54.

Folope, V., M. F. Hellot, J. M. Kuhn, P. Teniere, M. Scotte, and P. Dechelotte. 2008. Weight Loss and Quality of Life after Bariatric Surgery: A Study of 200 Patients after Vertical Gastroplasty or Adjustable Gastric Banding. *European Journal of Clinical Nutrition* 62(8): 1022–30.

Fort, Meredith P., Nadia Alvarado-Molina, Liz Peña, Carlos Mendoza Montano, Sandra Murillo, and Homero Martínez. 2013. "Barriers and Facilitating Factors for Disease Self-Management: a Qualitative Analysis of Perceptions of Patients Receiving Care for Type 2 Diabetes and/or Hypertension in San José, Costa Rica and Tuxtla Gutiérrez, Mexico." *BMC Family Practice* 14(1): 131.

Foucault, Michele. 1973. *The Birth of the Clinic: An Archaeology of Medical Perception.* A. Sheridan, trans. London: Tavistock Publications Ltd.

Foucault, Michele. 1977. *Discipline and Punish: The Birth of the Prison.* A. Sheridan, trans. New York: Pantheon Books.

Fraser, Lorna, Kimberly Edwards, Janet Cade, and Graham Clarke. 2010. "The Geography of Fast Food Outlets: A Review." *International Journal of Environmental Research and Public Health* 7: 2290–308. doi: 10.3390/ijerph7052290.

Freedland, Kenneth E., David C. Mohr, Karina W. Davidson, and Joseph E. Schwartz. 2011. "Usual and Unusual Care: Existing Practice Control Groups in Randomized Controlled Trials of Behavioral Interventions." *Psychosomatic Medicine* 73(4): 323–35.

Freedman, David S. 2011. Centers for Disease Control and Prevention, "Obesity– United States, 1988–2008." *Morbidity and Mortality Weekly Report* 60(1): 73–77.

Freire, Paulo. 1970. *Pedagogy of the Oppressed.* Translated by Myra Bergman Ramos. New York: Continuum.

Freire, Paulo. 2000. *Pedagogy of the Oppressed.* New York: Bloomsbury Publishing.

Friedman, Jonathan. 1994. *Cultural Identity and Global Process.* Thousand Oaks, CA: Sage.

Frisbie, Charlotte J. 1980. *Southwestern Indian Ritual Drama.* Albuquerque, NM: University of New Mexico Press.

Froehling, D. A., P. R. Daniels, K. F. Mauck, M. L. Collazo-Clavell, A. A. Ashrani, M. G. Sarr, T. M. Petterson, K. R. Bailey, and J. A. Heit. 2013. "Incidence of Venous Thromboembolism after Bariatric Surgery: a population-based cohort study." *Obesity Surgery* 23(11): 1874–79.

Fuster, Melissa, Robert F. Houser, Ellen Messer, Patricia Palma de Fulladolsa, Hedi Deman, and Odilia I. Bermudez. 2014. "Household-level Dietary Quality Indicator for Countries in Nutritional Transition: Application to Vulnerable Communities in El Salvador." *Public Health Nutrition* 17(3): 529–36.

Gailey, J. A. 2012. "Fat Shame to Fat Pride: Fat Women's Sexual and Dating Experiences." *Fat Studies: An Interdisciplinary Journal of Body Weight and Society* 1(1): 114–27.

Gallaher, Courtney M., John M. Kerr, Mary Njenga, Nancy K. Karanja, and Antoinette MGA WinklerPrins. 2013. "Urban Agriculture, Social Capital, and Food Security in the Kibera Slums of Nairobi, Kenya." *Agriculture and Human Values* 30(3): 389–404.

Gartin, M. 2012. "Food Deserts and Nutritional Risk in Paraguay." *American Journal of Human Biology* 24(3): 296–301.

Gawande, Atul, 2009. "The Cost Conundrum: What a Texas Town Can Teach Us About Health Care." *New Yorker*, June 1.

Gayle, Gordon D. 1996. "Bloody Beaches: The Marines at Peleliu." Washington, D.C.: Marine Corps Historical Center.

Gaziano, Thomas A., and Neha Pagidipati. 2013. "Scaling Up Chronic Disease Prevention Interventions in Lower- and Middle-Income Countries." *Annual Review of Public Health* 34(1): 317–335. doi:10.1146/annurev-publhealth-031912-114402.

Gerchow, Lauren, Barbara Tagliaferro, Allison Squires, Joey Nicholson, Stella M. Savarimuthu, Damara Gutnick, and Melanie Jay. 2014. "Latina Food Patterns in the United States." *Nursing Research* 63(3): 182–93.

Gewertz, Deborah, and Frederick Errington. 2010. *Cheap Meat: Flap Food Nations in the Pacific Islands*. Berkeley: University of California Press.

Giddens, Anthony. 1993. *Modernity and Self Identity: Self and Society in the Late Modern Age*. Redwood City, CA: Stanford University Press.

Gimlin, Debra. 2007. "What is Body Work? A Review of the Literature." *Sociology Compass* 1(1): 353–70.

Gimlin, Debra. 2002. *Body Work: Beauty and Self-Image in American Culture*. Santa Barbara, CA: University of California Press.

Giroux, Henry A. 2011. *On Critical Pedagogy*. New York: Bloomsbury Academic.

Glauber, Joseph. 2013. "The Growth of the Federal Crop Insurance Program 1990–2011." *American Journal Agricultural Economics* 95(2): 482–88. doi: 10.1093/ajae/aas091.

Gobato, Renata Cristina, Giseli Panigassi, and Juliana Pasti Villalba. 2010. "Identificação do Perfil de Usuários de um Restaurante Popular do Município de Campinas." *Revista Segurança Alimentar e Nutricional, Campinas* 17(2): 14–25.

Goffman, Erving. 1963. *Stigma: Notes on the Management of Spoiled Identity*. New York: Simon & Schuster, Inc.

Goodman, Alan H., and Thomas L. Leatherman. 1998. "Traversing the Chasm Between Biology and Culture: An Introduction." In *Building a New Biocultural Synthesis: Political-Economic Perspectives on Human Biology*, edited by Alan H. Goodman and Thomas L. Leatherman, 3–42. Ann Arbor, MI: University of Michigan Press.

Gordon, Andrew. 1993. "Contests for the Workplace." In *Postwar Japan as History*, edited by Andrew Gordon, 373–94. Berkeley: University of California Press.

Goryakin, Yevgeniy, Tim Lobstein, W. Philip T. James, and Marc Suhrcke. 2015. "The Impact of Economic, Political and Social Globalization on Overweight and Obesity in the 56 Low and Middle Income Countries." *Social Science and Medicine* 133: 67–76.

Gosman, G. G., W. C. King, B. Schrope, K. J. Steffen, G. W. Strain, A. P. Courcoulas, D. R. Flum, J. R. Pender, H. N. Simhan. 2010. "Reproductive Health of Women Electing Bariatric Surgery." *Fertility and Sterility* 94(4): 1426–31.

Government of Brazil. 2007. *III Conferência Nacional de Segurança Alimentar e Nutricional: Por um Desenvolvimento Sustentável com Soberania e Segurança Alimentar e Nutricional. Relatório Final* (Brasília: Government of Brazil).

G Government of Brazil. 2008. "Obesidade Atinge Mais da Metade da População Brasileira, Aponta Estudo (Brasília: Government of Brazil, August 8). Accessed January 2, 2015. http://www.brasil.gov.br/saude/2013/08/obesidade-atinge-mais- da-metade-da-populacao-brasileira-aponta-estudo.

overnment of Brazil. 2009. *Building Up the National Policy and System for Food and Nutrition Security: The Brazilian Experience* (Brasília: Government of Brazil).

Government of Brazil. 2011. *Alimentação Adequada e Saudável: Diretos de Todos. 4ª Conferência Nacional de Segurança Alimentar e Nutricional – Relatório Final: Declarações e Proposições* . Brasília: Government of Brazil).

Government of Brazil. 2015. "Restaurantes Populares." Accessed January 3, 2015. http://www.mds.gov.br/segurancaalimentar/equipamentos/restaurantespopulares.

Graff, Samantha, Dale Kunkel, and Seth Mermin. 2012. "Government Can Regulate Food Advertising To Children Because Cognitive Research Shows That It Is Inherently Misleading." *Health Affairs* 31(2): 392–98. doi: 10.1377/hlthaff.2011.0609.

Graham, H. 2012. "Smoking, Stigma and Social Class." *Journal of Social Policy* 41: 83–99.

Gray, C. M., K. Hunt, K. Lorimer, A. S. Anderson, M. Benzeval, and Wyke, S. 2011. "Words Matter: A Qualitative Investigation of Which Weight Status Terms are Acceptable and Motivate Weight Loss when used by Health Professionals." *BMC Public Health* 11: 513.

Greaney, Mary L., Faith D. Lees, Breanna Lynch, Linda Sebelia, and Geoffrey W. Greene. 2012. "Using Focus Groups to Identify Factors Affecting Healthful Weight Maintenance in Latino Immigrants." *Journal of Nutrition Education and Behavior* 44(5): 448–53.

Green, Lawrence W., M. Anne George, Mark Daniel, C. James Frankish, Carol P. Herbert, William R. Bowie, and Michel O'Neill. 2003. "Appendix C: Guidelines for Participatory Research in Health Promotion." In *Community-Based Participatory Research for Health*, edited by Meredith Minkler and Nina Wallerstein. San Francisco: Jossey-Bass Inc.

Greener, J., F. Douglas, and E. van Teijlingen. 2010. "More of the Same? Conflicting Perspectives of Obesity Causation and Intervention amongst Overweight People, Health Professionals and Policy Makers." *Social Science & Medicine* 70(7): 1042–9.

Greenhalgh, Susan. 2012. "Weighty Subjects: The Biopolitics of the U.S. War on Fat." *American Ethnologist* 39(3): 471–87.

Greenhalgh, Susan. and Megan A. Carney. 2014. "Bad Biocitizens?: Latinos and the US 'Obesity Epidemic'." *Human Organization* 73(3): 267–76.

Gremillion, H. 2005. "The Cultural Politics of Body Size." *Annual Review of Anthropology* 35: 13–32.

Grier, Sonya and Shiriki K. Kumanyika. 2008. "The Context for Choice: Health Implications of Targeted Food and Beverage Marketing to African Americans." *American Journal of Public Health* 98(9): 1616–29. doi: 10.2105/AJPH.2007.115626.

Griffith, David C. 2005. "'Rural Industry and Mexican Immigration and Settlement in North Carolina." In *New Destinations: Mexican Immigration in the United States*, edited by Victor Zúñiga and Ruben Hernández-Leon, 50–75. New York, Russell Sage.

Groven, K. S. 2014. "'They Think Surgery is Just a Quick Fix'." *International Journal of Qualitative Studies on Health and Well-Being* 9.

Groven, K. S., G. Engelsrud, and M. Råheim. 2013. "Changing Bodies, Changing Habits: Women's Experiences of Interval Training Following Gastric Bypass Surgery." *Health Care for Women International* 36(3):276–302

Groven, K. S., M. Råheim, and G. Engelsrud. 2013. "Dis-appearance and Dys-appearance Anew: living with excess skin and intestinal changes following weight loss surgery." *Medicine, Healthcare, and Philosophy* 16(3): 507–23.

Groven, K. S., M. Råheim, J. Braithwaite, and G. Engelsrud. 2013. "Weight Loss Surgery as a Tool for Changing Lifestyle?" *Medicine, Healthcare, and Philosophy* 16(4): 699–708.

Groven, K. S., G. Engelsrud, and M. Råheim. 2012. "Living with Bodily Changes after Weight Loss Surgery: Women's Experiences of Food and 'Dumping'." *Phenomenology & Practice* 6(1): 36–54.

Groven, K. S., M. Råheim, and G. Engelsrud. 2010. "My Quality of Life is Worse Compared to My Earlier Life": Living with chronic problems after weight loss surgery." *International Journal of Qualitative Studies on Health & Well-being* 5(4).

Hadley, Craig, and Deborah L. Crooks. 2012. "Coping and the Biosocial Consequences of Food Insecurity in the 21st Century." *American Journal of Physical Anthropology* 149(S55): 72–94.

Hagey, R. 1984. "The Phenomenon, the Explanations and the Responses: Metaphors Surrounding Diabetes in Urban Canadian Indians." *Social Science Medicine* 18(3): 265–272.

Hakim, C. 2010. "Erotic Capital." *European Sociological Review* 26(5): 499–518.

Haney-López, I.F. 1998. "Chance, Context, and Choice in the Social Construction of Race." In *The Latino/a Condition: A Critical Reader*. R. Delgado and J. Stefancic, eds. New York: New York University Press.

Harding, Kate and Marianne Kirby. 2009. *Lessons from the Fat-O-Sphere: Quit Dieting and Declare a Truce with your Body*. London: Penguin Group.

Hartroft, W. Stanley. 1960. "The Pathology of Obesity." *Bulletin of the New York Academy of Medicine* 36(5): 313–22.

Harvey, E. L. and A. J. Hill. 2001. "Health Professionals' Views of Overweight People and Smokers." *International Journal of Obesity & Related Metabolic Disorders* 25(8): 1253.

Hassan, M. Manzural. 2005. "Arsenic Poisoning in Bangladesh: Spatial Mitigation Planning with GIS and Public Participation." *Health Policy* 74(3): 247–60.

Hatzenbuehler, M. L., J. C. Phelan, and B. G. Link. 2013. "Stigma as a Fundamental Cause of Population Health Inequalities." *American Journal of Public Health* 103(5): 813–21.

Hatzenbuehler, M. L. and B. G. Link 2014. "Introduction to the Special Issue on Structural Stigma and Health." *Social Science and Medicine* 103: 1–6.

Hauff, L. E. and E. W. Demerath. 2012. "Body Image Concerns and Reduced Breastfeeding Duration in Primiparous Overweight and Obese Women." *American Journal of Human Biology* 24(3): 339–49.

Hayward, P. and Bright, J. A. 1997. "Stigma and Mental Illness: a Review and Critique." *Journal of Mental Health* 6(4): 345–54.

Hebl, M. R. and L. M. Mannix. 2003. "The Weight of Obesity in Evaluating Others: A Mere Proximity Effect." *Personality & Social Psychology Bulletin* 29(1): 28–38.

Henderson, L. C. 2010. "Divergent Models of Diabetes among American Indian Elders." *Journal of Cross-Cultural Gerontology* 25(4): 303–316.

Henrich, J., S. J. Heine and A. Norenzayan. 2010. "The Weirdest People in the World?" *Behavioral Brain Science* 33(2–3): 61–135.

Hergenrather, Kenneth C., Scott D. Rhodes, and Gerta Bardhoshi. 2009. "Photovoice as Community-Based Participatory Research: A Qualitative Review." *American Journal of Health Behavior* 33 (6): 686–98.

Herman, K. M., T. E. Carver, N. V. Christou, and R. E. Andersen. 2014. "Keeping the Weight Off: Physical Activity, Sitting Time, and Weight Loss Maintenance in Bariatric Surgery Patients 2 to 16 Years Post-surgery." *Obesity Surgery* February 28, 2014. [Epub ahead of print.]

Hernandez, Y., M. Zuniga-Escobar, M. Mora, and C. Gonzalez. 2011. "Needs Assessment of Eating Patterns of Costa Rican Overweight and Non-Overweight School-Aged Children: Implications for Childhood Obesity Prevention Efforts." *Journal of the American Dietetic Association* 111(9): A87.

Hilton, S., Patterson, C., and Teyhan, A. 2012. "Escalating Coverage of Obesity in UK Newspapers: The Evolution and Framing of the "Obesity Epidemic" from 1996 to 2010." *Obesity (Silver Spring)* 20(8): 1688–1695. doi: 10.1038/oby.2012.27.

Himmelgreen, David. 2013. "In Focus: Food Insecurity, Early Environment Adversity, and Long-Term Health". *Anthropology News* 54(12): e8–e22.

Himmelgreen, David, R. Pérez-Escamilla, D. Martinez, A. Bretnall, B. Eells, Y. Peng, and A. Bermúdez. 2004. "The Longer You Stay, the Bigger You Get: Length of Time and Language use in the U.S. are Associated with Obesity in Puerto Rican Women". *American Journal of Physical Anthropology* 125(1): 90–96.

Himmelgreen, David A., Nancy Romero Daza, Maribel Vega, Humberto Brenes Cambronero, and Edgar Amador. 2006. "'The Tourist Season Goes Down But Not the Prices.' Tourism and Food Insecurity in Rural Costa Rica." *Ecology of Food and Nutrition* 45(4): 295–321.

Himmelgreen, David A., Nancy Romero-Daza, Edgar Amador, and Cynthia Pace. 2012. "Tourism, Economic Insecurity, and Nutritional Health in Rural Costa Rica: Using Syndemics Theory to Understand the Impact of the Globalizing Economy at the Local Level." *Annals of Anthropological Practice* 36(2): 346–64.

Himmelgreen, David A., Allison Cantor, Sara Arias, and Nancy Romero Daza. 2013. "Using a Biocultural Approach to Examine Migration/Globalization, Diet Quality, and Energy Balance." *Physiology & Behavior* 134: 76–85

Himmelgreen, David A., Nancy Romero Daza, Allison Cantor, and Sara Arias-Steele. 2014. "Is the Cup Half-Empty or Half-Full?: Experiences and Perceptions of Food Security in the Face of Economic Transition in Rural Costa Rica." In *Women Redefining the Limits of the Food System and the Experience of Food Insecurity: Life off the Edge of the Table* edited by Janet Page Reeves. Lanham, MD: Lexington Press.

Hodge, D.R., G.E. Limb and T.L. Cross. 2009. Moving from Colonization toward Balance and Harmony: a Native American Perspective on Wellness." *Social Work* 54(3): 211–9.

Holston, James. 2008. *Insurgent Citizenship: Disjunctions of Democracy and Modernity in Brazil*. Princeton, NJ: Princeton University Press.

Holub, Christina K., John P. Elder, Elva M. Arredondo, Simón Barquera, Christina M. Eisenberg, Luz María Sánchez Romero, Juan Rivera, Felipe Lobero, and

Eduardo J. Simoes. 2013. "Obesity control in Latin American and U.S. Latinos: A Systematic Review." *American Journal of Preventive Medicine* 44(5): 529–37.

Hornby, G., and R. Lafaele. 2011. "Barriers to Parental Involvement in Education: an Explanatory Model." *Educational Review* 63(1): 37–52.

Horton, S. and J. C. Barker. 2010. "Stigmatized Biologies: Examining the Cumulative Effects of Oral Health Disparities for Mexican American Farmworker Children." *Medical Anthropology Quarterly* 24: 199–219.

Hruschka, Daniel J. (*forthcoming*) "From Thin to Fat and Back Again: A Dual Process Model of the Big Body Mass Reversal." In *Obesity, Upward Mobility, and Symbolic Capital in a Rapidly Changing World.* Santa Fe, NM: SAR Press.

Hruschka, Daniel J. 2012. "Do Economic Constraints on Food Choice Make People Fat? A Critical Review of Two Hypotheses for the Poverty-Obesity Paradox." *American Journal of Human Biology* 24(3): 277–85.

Hruschka, Daniel J., Alexandra Brewis, Amber Wutich, and B. Morin. 2011. "Shared Norms and Their Explanation for the Social Clustering of Obesity." *American Journal of Public Health* 101(Suppl 1): S295–300.

Huang, T. K., Harris, K. J., Lee, R. E., Nazir, N., Born, W. & Kaur, H. 2003. "Assessing Overweight, Obesity, Diet, and Physical Activity in College Students." *Journal of American College Health* 52(2): 83–86.

Hugo, G., and J. Franzon. 2006. "Child Obesity in South Australia." *Food, Culture & Society* 9(3): 299–316.

Hulens, M., G. Vansant, A.L. Claessens, R. Lysens, E. Muls, and R. Rzewnicki. 2002. "Health-Related Quality of Life in Physically Active and Sedentary Obese Women." *American Journal of Human Biology* 14(6): 777–85.

Humple, Nancy, Neville Owen, and Eva Leslie. 2003. "Environmental Factors Associated with Adults' Participation in Physical Activity, A Review." *American Journal of Preventive Medicine* 22(3): 188–99.

Hyland, Stanley E. 2005. "Community Building in the Twenty-First Century: Implications for Anthropologists." In *Community Building in the Twenty-First Century*, edited by Stanley E. Hyland, 219–32. Santa Fe, NM: School for Advanced Research Press.

Ichiho, Henry, Demei, Yorah, Kuartei, Stevenson, and Nia Aitaoto. 2013. "An Assessment of Non-Communicable Diseases, Diabetes, and Related Risk Factors in the Republic of Palau: A Systems Perspective." *Hawai'i Journal of Medicine and Public Health* 72(5): 98–105.

Ikeda, Nayu, Eiko Saito, Naoki Kondo, Manami Inoue, Shunya Ikeda, Toshihiko Satoh, Koji Wada, Andrew Stickley, Kota Katanoda, Tetsuya Mizoue, Hiroyasu Iso, Yoshihisa Fujino, Tomotaka Sobue, Shoichiro Tsugane, Mohsen Naghavi, Majid Ezzati, and Kenji Shibuya. 2011. "What Has Made the Population of Japan Healthy?" *The Lancet* 378 (9796): 1094–105.

Ikegami, Naoki, Byung-Kwang Yoo, Hideki Hashimoto, Masatoshi Matsumoto, Hiroya Ogata, Akira Babazono, Ryo Watanabe, Kenji Shibuya, Bong-Min Yang, Michael R. Reich, and Yasuki Kobayashi. 2011. "Japanese Universal Health Coverage: Evolution, Achievements, and Challenges." *The Lancet* 378(9796): 1106–15.

Ikegami, Naoki, and Akiko Maeda. 2014. "Overview." In *Universal Health Coverage for Inclusive and Sustainable Development: Lessons from Japan*, edited by Naoki Ikegami, 1–13. Washington, DC: The World Bank.

Institute of Medicine. 2012. *Accelerating Progress in Obesity Prevention: Solving the Weight of the Nation,* Washington, DC: National Academies Press. Accessed March 2, 2014. http://iom.edu/reports/2012/accelerating-progress-in-obesity- prevention.

Israel, Barbara A., Amy J. Schulz, Edith A. Parker, and Adam B. Becker. 2001. "Community-Based Participatory Research: Policy Recommendations for Promoting a Partnership Approach in Health Research." *Education for Health* 14(2): 182–97.

Israel Barbara, Amy Schulz, Edith Parker, and Adam Becker. 1998. "Review of Community-based Research: Assessing Partnership Approaches to Improve Public Health." *Annual Review of Public Health* 19: 173–202.

Israel, Barbara, Amy Schulz, Edith Parker, Adam Becker, Alex Allen, and Ricardo Guzman. 2003. "Critical Issues in Developing and Following Community Based Participatory Research Principles." In *Community Based Participatory Research for Health*, edited by Meredith Minkler and Nina Wallerstein, 53–76. San Francisco: John Wiley and Sons.

Israel, Barbara, Eugenia Eng, Amy Schulz, and Edith Parker, eds. 2013. *Methods for Community-Based Participatory Research for Health.* San Francisco: Jossey-Bass.

Jackson, Linda. 1992. *Physical Appearance and Gender: Sociobiological and Sociocultural Perspectives.* Albany, NY: State University of New York Press.

Jacoby, A. 1994. "Felt Versus Enacted Stigma: A Concept Revisited: Evidence from a Study of People with Epilepsy in Remission." *Social Science and Medicine* 38: 269–74.

Japan Ministry of Health, Labor, and Welfare (MHLW). 2007. *Basic Screening and Counseling program (Hyōjunteki na kenshin, hoken shidō purogramu).* MHLW Bureau of Health, Tokyo, Japan.

Javitt, J. C. and Y. P. Chiang. 2013. "Economic Impact of Diabetes". In *Diabetes in America,* edited by M. I. Harris. Bethesda, MD: National Institute of Diabetes and Digestive and Kidney Diseases.

Jensen, J. F., M. H. Petersen, T. B. Larsen, D. G. Jorgensen, H. N. Gronbaek, and J. Midtgaard. 2013. "Young Adult Women's Experiences of Body Image after Bariatric Surgery: A Descriptive Phenomenological Study." *Journal of Advanced Nursing* 70(5): 1138–49.

Joe, J. R. and S. Frishkopf. 2006. "I'm Too Young for This!": Diabetes and American Indian Children." In *Indigenous Peoples and Diabetes: Community Empowerment and Wellness*, edited by M. K. L. Ferreira and G. C. Lang. Durham, NC: Carolina Academic Press.

Johannes, R. E. 1981. *Words of the Lagoon: Fishing and Marine Lore in the Palau District of Micronesia.* Berkeley: University of California Press.

Johnson, James A., and Carleen H. Stoskopf. 2010. *Comparative health systems global perspectives.* Edited by James A. Johnson and Carleen H. Stoskopf. Jones and Bartlett Publishers: Sudbury, Mass.

Johnston, S. L. 2007. "Plate Half-Empty or Half-Full? Dietary Continuity and Change among the Blackfeet." Ecology of Food and Nutrition 46(5–6): 361–76.

Jones, E., A. Farina, A. Hastorf, H. Markus, D.T. Miller, and R. Scott. 1984. *Social Stigma: The Psychology of Marked Relationships*. New York: Freeman and Company.

Kahn, James G., Joshua S. Yang, and James S. Kahn. 2010. "'Mobile' Health Needs and Opportunities in Developing Countries." *Health Affairs* 29 (2):252–58.

Kanagawa Prefecture Electrical Appliance Health Insurance Union. 2010. *Metabolic Syndrome: Eat, Move, and Lose Body Fat*. (*Metaborikku shindorōmu: Tabete, ugoite, herasu naizō shibō*). Kanagawa Prefecture Electrical Appliance Health Insurance Union, Yokoyama, Japan.

Kandala, Ngianga-Bakwin, and Saverio Stranges. 2014. "Geographic Variation of Overweight and Obesity among Women in Nigeria: A Case for Nutritional Transition in Sub-Saharan Africa." *PloS One* 9(6): e101103

Kaufer-Horwitz, M., J. Martínez, L. M. Goti-Rodríguez, and H. Ávila-Rosas. 2006. "Association between Measured BMI and Self-Perceived Body Size in Mexican Adults." *Annals of Human Biology* 33(5–6): 536–45.

Keener, Dana, Kenneth Goodman, Amy Lowry, Susan Zaro, and Laura Kettel Khan. 2009. *Recommended Community Strategies and Measurements to Prevent Obesity in the United States: Implementation and Measurement Guide*. Atlanta, GA: U.S. Department of Health and Human Services, Centers for Disease Control and Prevention. Accessed August 24, 2015. http://www.cdc.gov/obesity/downloads/community_strategies_guide.pdf.

Kersh, Rogan. 2009. "The Politics of Obesity: A Current Assessment and the Look Ahead." *The Millbank Quarterly* 87(1): 295–316.

Kersh, Rogan, and James Morone. 2002. "The Politics of Obesity: Seven Steps to Government Action." *Politics and Public Health* 21(6): 142–53.

"Keyhole Garden Manual." 2009. *Center for Energy Studies*. Rice University's Baker Institute. Web. 30 July 2013. <http://bakerinstitute.org/programs/energyforum/publications/lesotho/khg%20card%20final%20ENGLISH.pdf/view?searchterm=Keyhole%20gardens>.

"Keyhole Gardens - an Innovative Organic Gardening Technique." 2010. Warm Earth (92): 28.

Kilpatrick, Kate. 2011. "Fighting Hunger in Brazil: Much Achieved, More to Do." *Oxfam Policy and Practice: Agriculture, Food and Land* 11(4): 89–96.

King, M., A. Smith and M. Gracey. 2009. "Indigenous Health Part 2: the Underlying Causes of the Health Gap." *Lancet* 374(9683): 76–85.

King, W. C., S. H. Belle, G. M. Eid, G. F. Dakin, W. B. Inabnet, J. E. Mitchell, E. J. Patterson, A. P. Courcoulas, D. R. Flum, W. H. Chapman, B. M. Wolfe and the Longitudinal Assessment of Bariatric Surgery Study. 2008. "Physical Activity Levels of Patients Undergoing Bariatric Surgery in the Longitudinal Assessment of Bariatric Surgery Study." *Surgery for Obesity and Related Diseases* 4(6): 721–28.

King, W. C., J. Y. Hsu, S. H. Belle, A. P. Courcoulas, G. M. Eid, D. R. Flum, J. E. Mitchell, J. R. Pender, M. D. Smith, K. J. Steffen, and B. M. Wolfe. 2012. "Pre- to postoperative Changes in Physical Activity: report from the Longitudinal Assessment of Bariatric Surgery-2 (LABS-2)." *Surgery for Obesity and Related Diseases* 8(5): 522–32.

Kingdon, John. 2003. *Agendas, Alternatives and Public Policies, 2nd edition.* New York: Longman.

Kittler, P. G., and K. Sucher. 2011. *Food and Culture.* 6th edition. Stamford, Connecticut: Cengage Learning.

Kitzinger, H. B., S. Abayev, A. Pittermann, B. Karle, H. Kubiena, A. Bohdjalian, F. B. Langer, G. Prager, and M. Frey. 2012. "The Prevalence of Body Contouring Surgery after Gastric Bypass Surgery." *Obesity Surgery* 22(1): 8–12.

Knowler, W. C. 2002. "Reduction in the Incidence of Type 2 Diabetes with Lifestyle Intervention or Metformin." *New England Journal of Medicine* 346(6): 393–403.

Knutsen, I. R., L. Terragni, and C. Foss. 2013. "Empowerment and Bariatric Surgery: Negotiations of Credibility and Control." *Qualitative Health Research* 23(1): 66–77.

Kottak, Conrad. 1999. "The New Ecological Anthropology." *American Anthropologist* 11(1): 23–35.

Krämer, Augustin. 1919. *Palau, vol.2.* Translated by Carmen Petrosian-Husa. [Online] Hamburg, L. Friedrichsen and Company. Reprinted on Etpisonmuseum.org, 2015. Accessed 31 July 2015. http://www.etpisonmuseum.org/kramer.html.

Krippendorff, K. 2012. *Content Analysis: An introduction to its methodology.* Thousand Oaks, CA: Sage.

Kuartei, Stevenson. 2011. "Declaration of the State of Health Emergency on Non-Communicable Diseases in Palau." Ministry of Health, Republic of Palau.

Kuartei, Stevenson. 2005. "Environment and Expression of the Thrifty Gene." *Pacific Health Dialogue* 12(1): 105–109.

Kulick, D., and A. Meneley. (eds). 2005. *Fat: The Anthropology of an Obsession.* London: Penguin Books.

Kumar, Gayathri S., Liping Pan, Sohyun Park, Seung Hee Lee-Kwan, Stephen Onufrak, and Heidi M. Blanck. 2014. "Sugar-sweetened Beverage Consumption among Adults—18 States, 2012." *Morbidity and Mortality Weekly Report* 63(32): 686–90.

Kunstler, James Howard. 1993. *The Geography of Nowhere: The Rise and Decline of America's Man-Made Landscape.* New York: Touchstone.

Labarthe, Darwin R., Dwayne Reed, Jacob A. Brody, and Reuel Stallones. 1973. "Health Effects of Modernization in Palau." *American Journal of Epidemiology* 98(3): 161–74.

Lamb-Parker, F., C. S. Piotrkowski, A. J. L. Baker, S. Kessler-Sklar, B. Clark, and L. Peay. 2001. "Understanding Barriers to Parent Involvement in Head Start: a Research-Community Partnership." *Early Childhood Research Quarterly* 16(1): 35–51.

Latner, J. D., D. S. Ebneter, and K. S. O'Brien. 2012. "Residual Obesity Stigma: An Experimental Investigation of Bias Against Obese and Lean Targets Differing in Weight-Loss History." *Obesity* 20(10): 2035–38.

Lavizzo-Mourey, R. 2009. "The Adolescent Obesity Epidemic." *Journal of Adolescent Health* 45(3): S6–7.

Leão, Marília, and Renato S. Maluf. 2012. *A Construção Social de um Sistema Público de Segurança Alimentar e Nutricional: A Experiência Brasileira* (Brasília: Government of Brazil).

Leatherman, Thomas L., and Alan Goodman. 2005. "Coca-Colonization of Diets in the Yucatan." *Social Science & Medicine* 61(4): 833–46.

Lee, J., and Bowen, N. 2006. "Parent Involvement, Cultural Capital, and the Achievement Gap among Elementary School Children." *American Educational Research Journal* 43: 193–218.

Lehnert, Thomas, Diana Sonntag, Alexander Konnopka, Steffi Riedel-Heller, and Hans-Helmut König, 2013. "Economic Costs of Overweight and Obesity." *Best Practice & Research: Clinical Endocrinology & Metabolism* 27: 105–15.

Levin, T. 2006. "Schizophrenia Should be Renamed to Help Educate Patients and the Public." *Journal of Social Psychiatry* 52(4): 324–31.

Lewis, S., Thomas, S.L., Hyde, J., Castle, D., Blood, R.W. and Komesaroff, P.A. 2010. "'I Don't Eat a Hamburger and Large Chips Every Day!' A Qualitative Study of the Impact of Public Health Messages about Obesity on Obese Adults." *BMC Public Health* 10(309): 1–9.

Li, J., and N. H. Hooker. 2010. "Childhood Obesity and Schools: Evidence from the National Survey of Children's Health". *Journal of School Health* 80(2): 96–103.

Lilleleht, E. 2002. "Progress and Power: Exploring the Disciplinary Connections Between Moral Treatment and Psychiatric Rehabilitation." *Philosophy, Psychiatry, and Psychology* 9(2): 167–182.

Lin B. H., C. L.Huang, and S. A. French. 2004. "Factors Associated with Women's and Children's Body Mass Indices by Income Status." *International Journal of Obesity*. 28: 536–42.

Lindberg, Nangel M., Victor J. Stevens, and Ruben O. Halperin. 2013. "Weight-loss Interventions for Hispanic Populations: The Role of Culture." *Journal of Obesity* 542736. doi: 10.1155/2013/542736.

Lindsay A. C., K. M. Sussner, K. Juhee, and S. Gortmaker. 2006. "The Role of Parents in Preventing Childhood Obesity." *Future of Children* 16(1): 169–86.

Link, B. G. 1987. "Understanding Labeling Effects in the Area of Mental Disorders: An Assessment of the Effects of Expectations of Rejection." *American Sociological Review* 52: 96–112.

Link, B. G. and J. C. Phelan. 2001. "Conceptualizing Stigma." *Annual Review of Sociology* 27: 363–385.

Link, B. G., F. T. Cullen, E. Struening, P. E. Shrout and B. P. Dohrenwend. 1989. "A Modified Labeling Theory Approach to Mental Disorders: An Empirical Assessment." *American Sociological Review* 54: 400–23.

Livingston, J. D., T. Milne, M. L. Fang, and E. Amari. 2012. "The Effectiveness of Interventions for Reducing Stigma Related to Substance Use Disorders: A Systematic Review." *Addiction* 107(1): 39–50.

Lock, Margaret. 1997. "Keeping Pressures Off the Japanese Health Care System: The Contribution of Middle-Aged Women." In *Containing Health Care Costs in Japan*, edited by Naoki Ikegami and John Creighton Campbell, 207–25. Ann Arbor: University of Michigan Press.

London, Jonathan, Jenny Saklar, Tara Mirel Zagofsky, and Ganlin Huang. 2011. "Collaboration, Participation and Technology: The San Juaquin Valley Cumulative

Health Impacts Project." *Gateways: International Journal of Community Research and Engagement* 4: 12–30.
Lund, E. M. and S. L. Miller. 2014. "Is Obesity Un-American?: Disease concerns bias implicit perceptions of national identity." *Evolution and Human Behavior* 35(4): 336–40.
Luque, John S. 2012. "Latinos Reduciendo el Diabetes (LaRED) Southeast Georgia Communities Project - Year 5 Evaluation Summary." Jiann-Ping Hsu College of Public Health, Georgia Southern University.
Luque, John S., Mondi Mason, Caludia Reyes-Garcia, Andrea Hinojossa, and Cathy D. Meade. 2011. "Salud es Vida: Development of a Cervical Cancer Education Curriculum for Promotora Outreach with Latina Farmworkers in Rural Southern Georgia." *American Journal of Public Health* 101(12): 2233–35.
Luque, John S., Carlos Reyes-Ortiz, Prasen Marella, Angelica Bowers, Viral Panchal, Lisa Anderson and Simone Charles. 2012. "Mobile Farm Clinic Outreach to Address Health Conditions among Latino Migrant Farmworkers in Georgia." *Journal of Agromedicine* 17(4): 386–97.
MacQueen, K. M., E. McLellan, K. Kay, and B. Milstein. 1998. "Codebook Development for Team-Based Qualitative Analysis." *Cultural Anthropology Methods* 10(2): 31–36.
Maddock, Jay. 2004. "The Relationship between Obesity and the Prevalence of Fast Food Restaurants: State-level Analysis." *American Journal of Health Promotion* 19(2): 137–43.
Maddox, G. L., K. W. Back, and V. R. Liederman. 1968. "Overweight as Social Deviance and Disability." *Journal of Health and Social Behavior* 9(4): 287–300.
Magdelano, R. Jr., E. A. Chaim, and E. R. Turato. 2010. "Understanding the Life Experiences of Brazilian Women after Bariatric Surgery: a Qualitative Study." *Obesity Surgery* 20(8): 1086–89.
Mainous, A. G., R. Baker, R. J. Koopman, S. Saxena, V. A. Diaz, C. J. Everett, and A. Majeed. 2007. "Impact of the Population at Risk of Diabetes on Projections of Diabetes Burden in the United States: An Epidemic on the Way." *Diabetologia* 50(5): 934–40. doi:10.1007/s00125-006-0528-5.
Margaret, Chan. 2011. "Non Communicable Diseases Damage Health, Including Economic Health." [Address]. The World Health Organization, Last Modified February 14, 2014. http://www.who.int/dg/speeches/2011/un_ncds_09_19/en/.
Martin, D. D. 2002. "From Appearance Tales to Oppression Takes: Frame Alignment and Organizational Identity." *Journal of Contemporary Ethnography* 31(2): 158–206.
Martin, Karen. 2008. *Consumer Health and Food Safety Report to the Pima County Board of Health.* Pima County Health Department, 9/24/08.
Martin, J. L. and M. George. 2006. "Theories of Sexual Stratification: Toward an Analytics of the Sexual Field and a Theory of Sexual Capital." *Sociological Theory* 24(2): 107–32.
Martin, Katie S., and Ann M. Ferris. 2007. "Food Insecurity and Gender are Risk Factors for Obesity." *Journal of Nutrition Education and Behavior* 39(1): 31–36.

Martin, M., A. Beekley, R. Kjorstad, and J. Sebesta. 2010. "Socioeconomic Disparities in Eligibility and Access to Bariatric Surgery: A National Population-based Analysis." *Surgery for Obesity and Related Diseases* 6(1): 8–15.

Mason, M. 2009. "Latinos Reduciendo el Diabetes (LaRED) Southeast Georgia Communities Project - Year 2 Evaluation Summary." Jiann-Ping Hsu College of Public Health, Georgia Southern University.

Mathule, Lineo M. 2009. "Interrelationships and Impact of Keyhole/Trench Gardens on Nutritional Status of HIV/AIDS Affected and Unaffected Beneficiaries in Lesotho." *Annals of Nutrition and Metabolism* 55: 250.

Mattingly, B. A., M. A. Stambush, and A. E. Hill. 2009. "Shedding the Pounds but not the Stigma: Negative Attributions as a Function of a Target's Method of Weight Loss." *Journal of Applied Biobehavioral Research* 14(3): 128–44.

Maupin, J. and A. Brewis. 2014. "Food Insecurity and Body Norms in Guatemalan Schoolchildren." *American Anthropologist* 116(2): 332–37.

Mayer, Jean. 1960. "Genetic Factors in Obesity." *Bulletin of the New York Academy of Medicine* 36(5): 323–43.

McCarthy, Michael. 2004. "Keyhole Gardening Saves Lives in World's Most Eroded Land." *The Independent*, December 27.

McCarty, C., J. L. Molina, C. Aguilar, and L. Rota. 2007. "A Comparison of Social Network Mapping and Personal Network Visualization." *Field Methods* 19(2), 145–162.

McClure, S. 2013. "'It's Just Gym': Physicality and identity among African American adolescent girls." Doctoral Dissertation. Case Western Reserve University.

McDonald's Corporation. "The Menu You Love and So Much More." Accessed December 30, 2014. http://www.mcdonalds.com/content/us/en/food/meal_bundles/dollar_menu.html

McGinnis, Michael, Jenifer Gootman, and Viveka Kraak. 2008. *Food Marketing to Children and Youth, Threat or Opportunity?* Washington, DC: National Academies Press.

McKenna, D., D. Selzer, M. Burchett, J. Choi, and S.G. Mattar. 2013. "Revisional bariatric surgery is more effective for improving obesity-related co-morbidities than it is for reinducing major weight loss." *Surgery for Obesity and Related Diseases* S1550–7289(13).

McLaughlin, H. 2009. "What's in a Name: 'Client', 'Patient', 'Customer', 'Consumer', 'Expert by Experience', 'Service User'—What't Next?" *British Journal of Social Work* 39: 1101–117.

McLemore, Jessica. 2015. "It Takes a Village to Feed a Child: Motives of Food Education in Japanese Elementary Schools." Senior thesis, Department of East Asian Studies, Princeton University.

McLeroy, Kenneth R., Daniel Bibeau, Allan Steckler, and Karen Glanz. 1988. "An Ecological Perspective on Health Promotion Programs." *Health Education & Behavior* 15(4): 351–77. doi: 10.1177/109019818801500401.

Meana, M. and L. Ricciardi. 2008. *Obesity Surgery: Stories of Altered Lives.* Reno, NV: University of Nevada Press.

Mechanick, J. I., A. Youdim, D. B. Jones, T. Garvey, D. Hurley, M. M. McMahon, L. J. Heinberg, R. Kuchner, T. D. Adams, S. Shikora, J. B. Dixon, S. Brethauer. 2013. "Clinical Practice Guidelines for the Perioperative Nutritional, Metabolic, and Nonsurgical Support of the Bariatric Surgery Patient—2013 Update: Cosponsored by American Association of Clinical Endocrinologists, The Obesity Society, and American Society for Metabolic & Bariatric Surgery." *Surgery for Obesity and Related Diseases* 9: 159–91.

Meiji Yasuda System Technology Corporation. 2009. *Good-bye Metabo! Health Support Text. (Sayonara! Metabo: kenkō shien tekisuto).* Health Care Total Support Enterprise, Tokyo, Japan.

Melby, Melissa K., and Wakako Takeda. 2014. "Lifestyle Constraints, Not Inadequate Nutrition Education, Cause Gap between Breakfast Ideals and Realities Among Japanese in Tokyo." *Appetite* 72(1): 37–49.

Mikecz, R. 2012. "Interviewing Elites: Addressing Methodological Issues." *Qualitative Inquiry* 18: 482.

Miller, D. P. Jr., J. G. Spangler, M. Z. Vitolins, S. W. Davis, E. H. Ip, G. S. Marion, and S. J. Crandall. 2013. "Are Medical Students Aware of their Anti-Obesity Bias?" *Academic Medicine* 88(7): 978–82.

Millman, Marcia. 1980. *Such a Pretty Face: Being Fat in America.* New York: W.W. Norton & Co. Inc.

Ministério de Desenvolvimento Social e Combate à Fome. 2015. "Restaurantes Populares" (Brasília: Government of Brazil). Accessed January 17, 2015. http://www.mds.gov.br/segurancaalimentar/equipamentos/restaurantespopulares.

Ministério de Desenvolvimento Social e Combate à Fome. *Manual Programa Restaurante Popular* (Brasília: Government of Brazil, 2004).

Ministério de Desenvolvimento Social e Combate à Fome. *Brasil Sem Miséria/Brazil Without Extreme Poverty Plan* (Brasília: Government of Brazil, 2012).

Ministério de Saúde. Guia Alimentar Para a População Brasileira. 2014. (Brasília: Government of Brazil). Accessed January 10, 2014. http://www.foodpolitics.com/wp-content/uploads/Brazils-Dietary-Guidelines_2014.pdf.

Minkler, Meredith. 2010. "Linking Science and Policy Through Community-Based Participatory Research to Study and Address Health Disparities." *American Journal of Public Health* 100(S1): S81–S87.

Mitka, Mike. 2005. "Does the Metabolic Syndrome Really Exist? Diabetes and Heart Disease Groups Spar Over Issue." *Journal American Medical Association* 294(16): 2010–13.

Moffat, Tina. 2010. The "Childhood Obesity Epidemic: Health Crisis or Social Construction?" *Medical Anthropology Quarterly* 24(1): 1–21.

Monteiro, Carlos A., and Geoffrey Cannon. 2012. "The Impact of Transnational "Big Food" Companies on the South: A View from Brazil." *PLoS Medicine* 9(7): e1001252.

Morris, Chad. 2011. "Assessing and Achieving Diversity of Participation in the Grant-Inspired Community-Based Public Health Coalition." *Annals of Anthropological Practice* 35(2): 43–65.

Morris, Chad, and John S. Luque. 2011. "Anthropological Insights on Effective Community-Based Coalition Practice: an Introduction." *Annals of Anthropological Practice* 35(2): 1–9.

Morris, Chad, Kelsey Collett, Jessica Deleconio, Caisee Foegle, and Nathan Sliwa. 2013. "Preliminary Report: Attitudes, Practices and Ideas Associated with

Nutrition and Food Security in Ngerbeched and Ngarchelong, Republic of Palau." Roanoke College.

Mourão, Luciana, and Anderson Macedo de Jesus. 2011. "Programa Bolsa Família: Uma Análise do Programa de Transferência de Renda Brasileiro." *Field Actions Science Reports. The Journal of Field Actions* Special Issue 3.

Mueser, K. T., S. M. Glynn, P. W. Corrigan and W. Baber. 1996. "A Survey of Preferred Terms for Users of Mental Health Services."*Psychiatric Services* 47(7): 760–61.

Mukherji, Nina, and Alfonso Morales. 2010. "Zoning for Urban Agriculture." *Zoning Practice* 27(3): 1–6.

Mundi, M. S., P. A. Lorentz, J. Swain, K. Grothe, and M. Collazo-Clavell. 2013. "Moderate Physical Activity as Predictor of Weight Loss After Bariatric Surgery." *Obesity Surgery* 23(10): 1645–49.

Murillo, Rosenda, Sandra S. Albrecht, Martha L. Daviglus, and Kiarri N. Kershaw. 2014. "The Role of Physical Activity and Sedentary Behaviors in Explaining the Association Between Acculturation and Obesity Among Mexican-American Adults." *American Journal of Health Promotion In-Press.* Accessed August 24, 2015. doi: 10.4278/ajhp.140128-QUAN-49

Murray, R. D. and S. Anzeljc. 2011. "Childhood Obesity in Practice." *Primary Care Reports* April 1.

Nadkarni, Nalini M., and Nathaniel T. Wheelwright, eds. 2000. *Monteverde: Ecology and Conservation of a Tropical Cloud Forest.* New York: Oxford University Press.

Nabhan, Gary Paul. 2002. *The Desert Smells Like Rain: A Naturalist in O'Odham Country*. Tucson: University of Arizona Press.

Nader, Laura. 1972. "Up the Anthropologist: Perspectives Gained from Studying Up." In *Reinventing Anthropology*, edited by Dell Hymes, 284–311. New York: Pantheon.

Namie, J. 2011. "Public Displays of Affection: Mothers, Children, and Requests for Junk Food." *Food Culture and Society* 14(3): 393–411.

Nanette L. Barkey, N. L., B. C. Campbell, and P. W. Leslie. 2001. "A Comparison of Health Complaints of Settled and Nomadic Turkana Men." *Medical Anthropology Quarterly* 15(3): 391–408.

National Center for Education Statistics. US Department of Education. Institute of Education Sciences, School Directory Information 2011–2012. Accessed April 1, 2014. http://nces.ed.gov/ccd/schoolsearch/index.asp.

National Diabetes Education Program. 2013. "Changing the Way Diabetes Is Treated: 15 Years." Accessed July 23, 2013. Available from: http://www.ndep.nih.gov/resources/ResourceDetail.aspx?ResId=420.

National Heart, Lung and Blood Institute. 2014. "Portion Distortion." Accessed December 31, 2014. http://www.nhlbi.nih.gov/health/educational/wecan/eat-right/portion-distortion.htm.

National Institute of Diabetes and Digestive and Kidney Diseases (NIDDK). 2014. *Talking with Patients about Weight Loss: Tips for Primary Care Providers*. National Institute of Health, U.S. Department of Health and Human Services.

Natvik, E., E. Gjengedal, and M. Råheim. 2013. "Totally changed, yet still the same: patients' lived experiences 5 years beyond bariatric surgery." *Qualitative Health Research* 23(9): 1202–14.

Neel, James V. 1962. "Diabetes Mellitus: A 'Thrifty' Genotype Rendered Detrimental by Progress." *American Journal of Human Genetics* 14: 352–53.

Neri, Marcelo. 2010. "The New Middle Class in Brazil: The Bright Side of the Poor." *Fundação Getúlio Vargas, Rio de Janeiro, Versão* 1.

Neri, Marcelo Cortes. 2014. "Good News for the Poor." *The Brazilian Economy* 2(10): 24–27.

New, Christin, Lan Xiao, and Jun Ma. 2013. "Acculturation and Overweight-Related Attitudes and Behavior among Obese Hispanic Adults in the United States." *Obesity* 21(11): 2396–404.

Nichols, Memorie, Aryeh D. Stein, and Judith Lupo Wold. 2014. "Health Status of Children of Migrant Farm Workers: Farm Worker Family Health Program, Moultrie, Georgia." *American Journal of Public Health* 104(2): 365–70.

Nichter, M. 2000. *Fat Talk: What Girls and their Parents Say about Dieting*. Cambridge: Harvard University Press.

Novick, A. 1997. "Stigma and AIDS: Three layers of damage." *Journal of the Gay and Lesbian Medical Association* 1: 53–60.

Nunez-Rivas, Hilda Patricia, Rafel Monge-Rojas, Hania León, and Marlen Roselló. 2003. "Prevalence of Overweight and Obesity among Costa Rican Elementary School Children." *Revista Panamericana de Salud Pública* 13(1): 24–32.

Obermeyer, C. M., S. Bott, P. Carrieri, M. Parsons, J. Pulerwitz, N. Rutenberg, and A. Sarna. 2009. "HIV Testing, Treatment and Prevention: generic tools for operational research." Geneva: World Health Organization.

O'Brien, Matthew J., Victor A. Alos, Adam Davey, Angeli Bueno, and Robert C. Whitaker. 2014. "Acculturation and the Prevalence of Diabetes in US Latino Adults, National Health and Nutrition Examination Survey 2007–2010." *Preventing Chronic Disease* 11: 140–42. doi: 10.5888/pcd11.140142

Offer, Avner, Rachel Pechey, and Stanley Ulijaszek. 2010. "Obesity under Affluence Varies by Welfare Regimes: The Effect of Fast Food, Insecurity, and Inequality." *Economics & Human Biology* 8(3): 297–308. doi: 10.1016/j.ehb.2010.07.002.

Ogden, Cynthia L., Margaret D. Carroll, Brian K. Kit., and Katherine M. Flegal. 20.14. "Prevalence of Childhood and Adult Obesity in the United States, 2011–2012." *Journal of the American Medical Association* 311(8): 806–14.

Orbach, Susie. 1978. *Fat is a Feminist Issue*. London: Arrow.

Organization for Economic Cooperation and Development. 2013. "Overweight and Obesity." In *OECD Factbook 2013: Economic, Environmental and Social Statistics*. OECD Publishing. Accessed August 21, 2015. DOI: 10.1787/factbook-2013-en

Ohnuki-Tierney, Emiko, 1984. *Illness and Culture in Contemporary Japan: An Anthropological View*. Cambridge: Cambridge University Press.

Oliver, J. Eric. 2006. *Fat Politics: The Real Story Behind America's Obesity Epidemic*. New York: Oxford University Press.

Omura, E. 2006. "Mino-Miijim's "Good Food for the Future": Beyond Culturally Appropriate Diabetes Programs, in Indigenous Peoples." In *Diabetes: Community*

Empowerment and Wellness, edited by M. K. L. Ferreira and G. C. Lang. Durham, NC: Carolina Academic Press.
Oregon Health Authority. 2012. "Oregon Overweight, Obesity, Physical Activity and Nutrition Facts." Accessed August 24, 2015. https://public.health.oregon.gov/PreventionWellness/PhysicalActivity/Documents/Oregon_PANfactst_2012.pdf.
Palmer, D. and J.J. Kronenfeld. 2012. *Social and Health Changes Following Bariatric Surgery*. Paper presented at the American Sociological Association Annual Meeting, Colorado Convention Center and Hyatt Regency, Denver, CO. Accessed online January 8, 2014. http://citation.allacademic.com/meta/p562991_index.html.
Parker, R., P. Aggleton, K. Attawell, J. Pulerwitz, and L. Brown. 2002. *HIV/AIDS-related stigma and discrimination: a conceptual framework and an agenda for action*. Washington, DC: Population Council, Horizons Program.
Patton, Michael Quinn. 1997. *Utilization Focused Evaluation: The New Century Text*. Thousand Oaks, CA: Sage Publications.
Penn, D. and A. Drummond. 2001. "Politically Correct Labels and Schizophrenia: A Rose by Any Other Name?" *Schizophrenia Bulletin* 27(2): 197–203.
Penney, Tarra L., and Sara F. L. Kirk. 2015. "The Health at Any Size Paradigm of Obesity: Missing Empirical Evidence May Help Push the Reframing Obesity Debate Forward." *American Journal of Public Health* 105(5): 38–42.
Perez-Escamilla, Rafael. 2011."Acculturation, Nutrition, and Health Disparities in Latinos." *American Journal of Clinical Nutrition* 93(5): 1163S–67S.
Pérez-Escamilla, Rafael. 2002. "The Childhood Obesity Epidemic in the USA: Epidemiology, Causes, and Solutions." *Nutritional Anthropology* 25(1): 29–35.
Pérez-Escamilla, R., D. Himmelgreen, H. Bonello, A. González, and L. Haldeman. 2001. "Nutrition Knowledge, Attitudes, and Behaviors among Latinos in the USA: Influence of language." *Ecology of Food and Nutrition* 40(4): 321–45.
Perez, Lilian G., Elva M. Arredondo, John P. Elder, Simón Barquera, Brian Nagle, and Christina K. Holub. 2013. "Evidence-based Obesity Treatment Interventions for Latino adults in the U.S.: A Systematic Review." *American Journal of Preventive Medicine* 44(5): 550–60.
Pérez, Wilton, Elmer Zelaya Blandón, Lars-Ake Persson, Rodolfo Peña, and Carina Kallestal. 2012. "Progress towards Millennium Development Goal 1 in Northern Rural Nicaragua: Findings from a Health and Demographic Surveillance Site." *International Journal of Equity and Health* 11(1): 43.
Perkins, Sue, and Robyn Lynn. 2000. "A Women's Community Garden: A Small Step towards a Future of Peace?" *Women Against Violence: An Australian Feminist Journal* 9: 74.
Pescosolido, B.A., J. L. Martin, A. Lang, and S. Olafsdottir. 2008. "Rethinking Theoretical Approaches to Stigma: A framework integrating normative influences on stigma." *Social Science & Medicine* 67(3): 431–40.
Pike, I. L. 2004. "The Biosocial Consequences of Life on the Run: A Case Study from Turkana District, Kenya." *Human Organization* 63(2): 221–235.
Pike, I. L. 2013. "In Focus: Remembered Hunger in an Increasingly Obese World." *Anthropology News* 54(12): e8–e22.

Pobocik, Rebecca, G. M. Heathcote, J. B. Spiers, and C. T. Otto. 2009. "Nutritional and Anthropometric Assessment of a Sample of Pregnant Women and Young Children in Palau." *Asia Pacific Journal of Clinical Nutrition* 9(2): 102–14.

Pomeranz, J. 2008. "A Historical Analysis of Public Health, the Law, and Stigmatized Social Groups: The Need for Both Obesity and Weight Bias Legislation." *Obesity* 16(2): S93–S103.

Popkin, Barry. 2004. "The Nutrition Transition and the Global Shift Towards Obesity." *Diabetes Voice* 49(3): 38–40.

Popkin, Barry M., Linda S. Adair, and Shu Wen Ng. 2012. "Global Nutrition Transition and the Pandemic of Obesity in Developing Countries." *Nutrition Reviews* 70(1): 3–21.

Poveda, A., M. E. Ibáñez, and E. Rebato. 2014. "Obesity and Body Size Perceptions in a Spanish Roma Population." *Annals of Human Biology* 41(5): 428–35.

Powdermaker, Hortense. 1960. "An Anthropological Approach to the Problem of Obesity." *Bulletin of the New York Academy of Medicine* 36(5): 286–95.

Powell, Lisa M., Sandy Slater, Donka Mirtcheva, Yanjun Bao, and Frank J. Chaloupka. 2007. "Food Store Availability and Neighborhood Characteristics in the United States." *Preventive Medicine* 44(3): 189–95.

Prasad, C., J. A. Batsis, F. Lopez-Jimenez, M. M. Clark, V. K. Somers, M. G. Sarr, and M. L. Collazo-Clavell. 2012. "Risk Perception of Obesity and Bariatric Surgery in Patients Seeking Treatment for Obesity." *European Journal of Preventative Cardiology* 21(6): 692–703.

Proper, Karin, Amika S. Singh, Willem van Mechelen, and Mai J. M. Chinapaw. 2011. "Sedentary Behaviors and Health Outcomes Among Adults, A Systematic Review of Prospective Studies." *American Journal of Preventive Medicine* 40(2): 174–82.

Puhl, R., J. L. Peterson and J. Luedicke. 2013. "Motivating or Stigmatizing? Public Perceptions of Weight-Related Language Used by Health Providers." *International Journal of Obesity* 37(4): 612–19.

Puhl, R. M., J. L. Peterson and J. Luedicke. 2011. "Parental Perceptions of Weight Terminology that Providers Use with Youth." *Pediatrics* 128(4): 786–93.

Puhl, R. M. and C. A. Heuer. 2009. "The Stigma of Obesity: A Review and Update." *Obesity* 17(5): 941–64.

Ramirez, Amelie G., Kipling J. Gallion, Cliff E. Despres, and Rebecca T. Adeigbe. 2013. "SaludAmerica!: A National Research Network to Build the Field and Evidence to Prevent Latino Childhood Obesity." *American Journal of Preventive Medicine* 44(Suppl 3): S178–85.

Raphael, D., A. Curry-Stevens and T. Bryant. 2008. "Barriers to Addressing the Social Determinants of Health: Insights from the Canadian Experience." *Health Policy* 88(2–3): 222–35.

Rede Xique Xique. "Instituição." Accessed January 2, 2015. http://redexiquexique.blogspot.com.br/p/instituicao.html.

Redman, Eric. 1973. *The Dance of Legislation.* New York: Simon and Schuster.

Reed, Frankie A. 2011. "Compact of Free Association with the Republic of Palau: Assessing the 15-year Review: Statement before Senate Committee on Energy and

Natural Resources." Accessed online August 27, 2015. http://www.state.gov/p/eap/rls/rm/2011/06/166289.htm.

Reich, Michael R., Naoki Ikegami, Kenji Shibuya, and Keizo Takemi. 2011. "50 Years of Pursuing a Healthy Society in Japan." *The Lancet* 378(9796): 1051–53.

Reid, T. R., 2009. *The Healing of America: The Global Quest for Better, Cheaper, and Fairer Health Care*. New York: Penguin Press.

Reischer, E. and K. S. Koo. 2004. "The Body Beautiful: Symbolism and Agency in the Social World." *Annual Review of Anthropology* 33: 297–317.

Rhee, Jinnie J., Josiemer Mattei, and Hannia Campos. 2012. "Association between Commercial and Traditional Sugar-Sweetened Beverages and Measures of Adiposity in Costa Rica." *Public Health Nutrition* 15(8): 1347–54.

Ro, Annie, and Nancy Fleischer. 2014. "Changes in Health Selection of Obesity among Mexican Immigrants: A Binational Examination." *Social Science & Medicine* 123: 114–24.

Robinson, Tanya. 2008. "Applying the Socio-Ecological Model to Improving Fruit and Vegetable Intake among Low-Income African Americans." *Journal of Community Health* 33: 395–406.

Rogge, M. M., M. Greenwald, and A. Golden. 2004. «Obesity, Stigma, and Civilized Oppresion." *Advances in Nursing Science* 27(4): 301–15.

Romero-Daza, Nancy; David. A. Himmelgreen, Charlotte A. Noble, and David Turkon. 2009. "Dealing with the Global Food Crisis in Local Settings: Non-intensive Agriculture in Lesotho, Southern Africa." *NAPA Bulletin* 32(1): 23–41.

Rothblum, E. D. 1992. "The Stigma of Women's Weight: Social and Economic Realities." *Feminism & Psychology* 2: 61–73.

Rothblum, E. D. and S. Solovay (eds). 2009. *The Fat Studies Reader*. New York: New York University.

Rudd Center for Food Policy and Obesity. 2014. "How to Talk About "Weight" with Your Overweight and Obese Patients." In *Improving Provider-Patient Interactions*. Rudd Center for Food Policy and Obesity, Yale University.

Rudd Center for Food Policy and Obesity. 2013. "Fast Food Facts: 2013, Measuring Progress In Nutrition and Marketing to Children and Teens." Accessed May 26, 2015. http://www.fastfoodmarketing.org/

Rueda-Clausen, Christian F., Federico A. Silva, and Patricio López-Jaramillo. 2008. "Epidemic of overweight and obesity in Latin America and the Caribbean." *International Journal of Cardiology* 125 (1): 111–112. doi:10.1016/j.ijcard.2006.12.092.

Sabin, J. A., M. Marini, and B. A. Nosek. 2012. "Implicit and Explicit Anti-Fat Bias among a Large Sample of Medical Doctors by BMI, Race/Ethnicity and Gender." *PLoS ONE* 7(11): e48448.

Saguy, Abigail. 2013. *What's Wrong with Fat?* Oxford, UK: Oxford University Press.

Saguy, Abigail. and R. Almeling. 2007. "Fat in the Fire? Science, the News Media, and the "Obesity Epidemic"." *Sociological Forum* 23(1): 53–83.

Saksvig, B. I. 2005. "A Pilot School-Based Healthy Eating and Physical Activity Intervention Improves Diet, Food Knowledge, and Self-Efficacy for Native Canadian Children." *Journal of Nutrition* 135(10): 2392–98.

Salter, Jonathan, Cam Campbell, Murray Journeay, anfd Stephen Sheppard. 2009. "The Digital Workshop: Exploring the Use of Interactive and Immersive Visualisation Tools in Participatory Planning." *Journal of Environmental Management* 90(6): 2090–101.

Santos, Martha S. 2014. "Recreating Patriarchy in Northeast Brazil:." Luso-Brazilian Review 51(2): 150–69.

Satinsky, S., B. Dennis, M. Reece, S. Sanders, and S. Bardzell. 2013. "My "Fat Girl Complex": A Preliminary Investigation of Sexual Health and Body Image in Women of Size." *Culture, Health & Sexuality* 15(6): 710–25.

Satterfield, Dawn. 2007. "So That the People May Live (Hecel Lena Oyate Ki Nipi Kte): Lakota and Dakota Elder Women as Reservoirs of Life and Keepers of Knowledge about Health Protection and Diabetes Prevention." *Journal of Health Disparities Research and Practice* 1(2): 1–28.

Satterfield, Dawn and P. T. Reid. 2003."'We Make the Road by Walking" with the People." *Diabetes Spectrum* 16(4): 213–215.

Satterfield, Dawn, Marla Burns, and Dave Baldridge. 2008. "Respecting Science and Community Wisdom: Adapting the Essential Public Health Services as a Framework."

Schensul, Jean J. 2005. "Strengthening Communities through Research Partnerships for Social Change': Perspectives from the Institute for Community Research." In *Community Building in the Twenty-First Century*, edited by Stanley E. Hyland, 191–218. Santa Fe, NM: School for Advanced Research Press.

Schiller, J. S., J. W. Lucas, B. W. Ward, and J. A. Peregoy. 2012. "Summary Health Statistics for U.S. adults: National Health Interview Survey, 2010." *Vital Health Statistics* 10(252): 1–207.

Schilling, Joseph and Leslie Linton. 2005. "Public Health Roots of Zoning." *American Journal of Preventive Medicine* 28(2) Supplement 2: 96.

Schlossberg, Marc, and Elliot Shuford. 2005. "Delineating 'Public' and 'Participation' in PPGIS." *URISA Journal* 16(2): 15–26.

Schupp, Justin L., and Jeff S. Sharp. 2012. "Exploring the Social Bases of Home Gardening." *Agriculture and Human Values* 29(1): 93–105.

Schur, Sylvia. 1960. "Simplified Diet Planning for the Patient." *Bulletin of the New York Academy of Medicine* 36(6): 399–406.

Schuster, Donald R. 2009. "The Republic of Palau and its Compact, 1995–2009." *The Journal of Pacific History* 44(3): 325–32.

Schwartz, M. B., L. R. Vartanian, B. A. Nosek, and K. D. Brownell. 2006. "The Influence of one's own Body Weight on Implicit and Explicit Anti-Fat Bias." *Obesity* 14(3): 440–47.

Seiden, A., N. L. Hawley, D. Schulz, S. Raifman, and S. T. McGarvey. 2012. "Long-Term Trends in Food Availability, Food Prices, and Obesity in Samoa." *American Journal of Human Biology* 24(3): 286–95.

Sharma, V., D. Whitney, S. S. Kazarian and R. Manchanda. 2000. "Preferred Terms for Users of Mental Health Services Among Service Providers and Recipients." *Psychiatric Services* 51(2): 203–209.

Shildrick, M. and J. Price. 1998. *Vital Signs: Feminist Reconfigurations of the Bio/logical Body*. Scotland: Edinburgh University Press.

Shillington, Laura J. 2013. "Right to Food, Right to the City: Household Urban Agriculture, and Socionatural Metabolism in Managua, Nicaragua." *Geoforum* 44: 103–11.

Shore, Cris, and Susan Wright. 1997. *Anthropology of Policy.* London: Routledge.

Silva, Luiz Inácio Lula de. 2011. "The Zero Hunger Project: A Proposal for a Food Security Policy in Brazil," in *The Fome Zero (Zero Hunger) Program: The Brazilian Experience* edited by José Graziano da Silva, Mauro Eduardo Del Grossi and Caio Galvão de França, 13–15. Brasília: FAO.

da Silva, S.S.P. and Â.d.C. Maia. 2013. "Patients' experiences after bariatric surgery: a qualitative study at 12-month follow-up." *Clinical Obesity* 3: 185–93.

da Silva, S. S. P. and Â. d. C. Maia. 2012. "Obesity and Treatment Meanings in Bariatric Surgery Candidates: A Qualitative Study." *Obesity Surgery* 22(11): 1714–22.

Simon, Jessica. 2014. "Food Security: Beyond Calories." *Journal of International Affairs* 67(2): 201.

Simon, P. 2012. "Charity's 'Keyhole' Gardens are Changing Lives in War-Torn State." Western Morning News, June 18.

Simpkins, S. D., D. R. Schaefer, C. D. Price, and A. E. Vest. 2013. "Adolescent Friendships, BMI, and Physical Activity: Untangling Selection and Influence Through Longitudinal Social Network Analysis." *Journal of Research on Adolescence* 23(3): 537–49.

Singer, Merrill. 2014. "Following the Turkey Tails: Neoliberal Globalization and the Political Ecology of Health." *Journal of Political Ecology,* 21: 436–51.

Singer, Merrill, Nicola Bullied, and Bayla Ostrach. 2012. "Syndemics and Human Health: Implications for Prevention and Intervention." *Annals of Anthropological Practice* 36(2): 205–11.

Singh, Gopal, Mohammad Siahpush, Robert A. Hiatt, and Lava R. Timsina. 2011. "Dramatic increases in obesity and overweight prevalence and Body Mass Index among ethnic-immigrant and social class groups in the United States, 1976-2008." *Journal of Community Health* 36(1): 94–110.

Sistema OCB. 2013. "Cooperativismo Agropecuário." (Brasília: OCB Sistema, August 25). Accessed January 2, 2015. http://www.agricultura.gov.br/arq_editor/file/camaras_tematicas/Insumos_agropecuarios/71RO/app_ocb.pdf.

Sjöström, L., A. K. Lindroos, M. Peltonen, J. Torgerson, C. Bouchard, B. Carlsson, S. Dahlgren, B. Larsson, K. Narbro, C. D. Sjöström, M. Sullivan, and H. Wedel. 2004. "Lifestyle, Diabetes, and Cardiovascular Risk Factors 10 Years after Bariatric Surgery." *New England Journal of Medicine* 351(26): 2683–93.

Smith, Brendan T., Peter M. Smith, Sam Harper, Douglas G. Manuel, and Cameron A. Mustard. 2014. "Reducing Social Inequalities in Health: the Role of Simulation Modelling in Chronic Disease Epidemiology to Evaluate the Impact of Population Health Interventions." *Journal of Epidemiology and Community Health* 68: 6.

Smith, C. A., K. Schmoll, J. Konik and S. Oberlander. 2007. "Carrying Weight for the World : Influence of Weight Descriptors on Judgments of Large-Sized Women." *Journal of Applied Social Psychology* 37: 989–1006.

Smith, C. Scott, Magdalena Morris, William Hill, Chris Francovich, Juliet McMullin, Leo Chavez, and Caroline Rhoads. 2004. "Cultural Consensus Analysis as a

Tool for Clinic Improvements." *Journal of General Internal Medicine* 19(5 Pt 2): 514–18.

Snell, Bradford C. 1974. "American Ground Transport: A Proposal for Restructuring the Automobile, Bus, and Rail Industries." Testimony presented to the Subcommittee on Antitrust and Monopoly of the Committee on the Judiciary, US Senate. Accessed January 5, 2015. http://libraryarchives.metro.net/DPGTL/testimony/1974_statement_bradford_c_snell_s1167.pdf.

Soares, Fábio Veras, Rafael Perez Ribas, and Rafael Guerreiro Osório. 2010. "Evaluating the Impact of Brazil's Bolsa Familia: Cash Transfer Programs in Comparative Perspective." *Latin American Research Review* 45(2): 173–90.

Sobal, Jeffrey. 1998. "Cultural Comparison Research Designs in Food, Eating, and Nutrition." *Food Quality and Preference* 9(6): 385–92.

Sobal, Jeffrey and D. Maurer (eds). 1999. *Interpreting Weight: The Social Management of Fatness and Thinness*. Berlin: Walter de Gruyter, Inc.

Sonoran Institute. 2014. Mission and Vision. Accessed December 30, 2014. http://www.sonoraninstitute.org/about-us/missionandvision.html.

Speakman, J. R. 2008. "Thrifty vs. Drifty Gene Theory of Obesity. *International Journal of Obesity* 32: 1611–15.

Stafford, M. C. and R. R. Scott. 1986. "Stigma, Deviance, and Social Control." In *The Dilemma of Difference: A Multidisciplinary View of Stigma*. S.C. Ainlay, G. Becker, and L. M. Coleman, eds. New York: Springer.

State of São Paulo. "Bom Prato." Accessed January 3, 2015. http://www.desenvolvimentosocial.sp.gov.br/portal.php/bomprato

St. Clair, David J. 1981. "The Motorization and Decline of Urban Public Transit, 1935–1950." *The Journal of Economic History* 41(3): 579–600. doi: 10.1017/S002205070004434X.

Steinberg, Sheila Lakshmi, Steven Steinberg, Jennifer Kauffman, and Josef Eckert. ND. "Public Participation GIS Research and Agricultural Farmworkers in California." Accessed August 24, 2015. http://proceedings.esri.com/library/userconf/proc08/papers/papers/pap_1703.pdf.

Story, Mary, Karen Kaphingst, Ramona Robinson-O'Brien, and Karen Glanz. 2008. "Creating Healthy Food and Eating Environments: Policy and Environmental Approaches." *Annual Review of Public Health* 29: 253–72.

Strand, Kerry. 2003. "Community-Based Research and Higher Education Principles and Practices." San Francisco: Jossey-Bass.

Strauss, Anselm, and Juliet Corbin. 1994. "Grounded Theory Methodology." *Handbook of Qualitative Research*, 273–85. Thousand Oaks, CA: Sage Publications.

Sudan, R., D. Winegar, S. Thomas, and J. Morton. 2014. "Influence of Ethnicity on the Efficacy and Utilization of Bariatric Surgery in the USA." *Journal of Gastrointestinal Surgery* 18(1): 130–36.

Suginami Ward Board of Education. 2012. "Suginami no gakkō kyūshoku no ayumi (The Historical Path of School Lunches in Suginami Ward)." Tokyo, Japan: Suginami Ward Board of Education Publishing (Suginami Kyōiku Iinkai Hakkō).

Suter, M., J. M. Calmes, A. Paroz, S. Romy, and V. Giusti. 2009. "Results of Roux-en-Y Gastric Bypass in Morbidly Obese vs. Superobese Patients: Similar Body

Weight Loss, Correction of Comorbidities, and Improvement of Quality of Life." *Archives of Surgery* 144(4): 312–18.

Swanson, C. M., L. R. Roust, K. Miller, and J. A. Madura II. 2012. "What Every Hospitalist Should Know about the Post-bariatric Surgery Patient." *Journal of Hospital Medicine* 7(2): 156–63.

Swift, J. A., E. Choi, R. M. Puhl and C. Glazebrook. 2013. "Talking about Obesity with Clients: Preferred Terms and Communication Styles of U.K. Pre-Registration Dieticians, Doctors, and Nurses." *Patient Education and Counseling* 91(2): 186–91.

Swinburn, Boyd, Garry Egger, and Fezeela Raza. 1999. "Dissecting Obesogenic Environments: The Development and Application of a Framework for Identifying and Prioritizing Environmental Interventions for Obesity." *Preventive Medicine* 29: 563–70.

Tailor, A. and J. Ogden. 2009. "Avoiding the Term "Obesity": an Experimental Study of the Impact of Doctors' Language on Patients' Beliefs." *Patient Education and Counseling* 76: 260–74.

Talen, Emily. 2000. "Bottom-Up GIS." *Journal of the American Planning Association* 66(3): 279–95.

Talukdar, J. 2012. "Thin but not Skinny: Women Negotiating the "never too thin" Body Ideal in Urban India." *Women's Studies International Forum* 35: 109–18.

Tapias, M. 2006. "Emotions and the Intergenerational Embodiment of Social Suffering in Rural Bolivia." *Medical Anthropology Quarterly* 20(3): 399–415.

Taylor, Nicole. 2015. "'Guys, She's Humongous!': Gender and Weight Based Teasing in Adolescence." *Journal of Adolescent Research* 26(2): 178–99.

Taylor, Nicole. 2006. "Constructing Gendered Identities through Discourse: Body Image, Exercise, Food Consumption, and Teasing Practices among Adolescents. PhD Dissertation. Tucson: University of Arizona.

Teague, Michael L, Sara L. C. Mackenzie, and David M. Rosenthal. 2013. *Your health today*: McGraw-Hill.

Thaler, Richard H., and Cass R. Sunstein. 2008. *Nudge: Improving Decisions About Health, Wealth, and Happiness*. New York: Penguin Books.

Throsby, K. 2008. "Happy Re-birthday: Weight-loss Surgery and the 'New Me'." *Body & Society* 14(1): 117–33.

Trainer, Sarah. 2013. "Local Interpretations of Global Trends: Body Concerns and Self-Projects Enacted by Young Emirati Women." *Doctoral Dissertation*. University of Arizona.

Trainer, Sarah, Alexandra Brewis, Daniel Hruschka, and Deborah Williams. 2015. "Translating Obesity: Navigating the Front Lines of the 'War on Fat'." *American Journal of Human Biology* 27(1): 61–68.

Trainer, Sarah, Alexandra Brewis, Deborah Williams and Jose Rosales Chavez. 2015. "Obese, Fat, or Big? Youth Deployment of and Reactions to Weight Terms." *Human Organization* 74: 3.

Tucci S. A., Boyland E. J., Halford J. C. G., Harrold J. A. 2013. "Stigmatisation of a Formerly Obese Young Female." *Obesity Facts* 6(5): 433–42.

Turner, Anne M., Elizabeth D. Liddy, Jana Bradley, and Joyce A. Wheatley. 2005. "Modeling Public Health Interventions for Improved Access to the Gray Literature." *Journal of the Medical Library Association* 93(4): 487–94.

Ulijaszek, Stanley J. 2007. "Frameworks of Population Obesity and the use of Cultural Consensus Modeling in the Study of Environments Contributing to Obesity." *Economics & Human Biology* 5(3): 443–57.

UNICAFES. Accessed January 2, 2015. http://unicafes.org.br/.

United States Census Bureau. 2013a. "State and County QuickFacts." Accessed August 2, 2015. http://quickfacts.census.gov/qfd/states/04/04019.html.

United States Census Bureau. 2013b. "State and County QuickFacts." Accessed August 2, 2015. http://factfinder.census.gov/faces/tableservices/jsf/pages/productview.xhtml?src=bkmk.

United States Census Bureau. 2008. "Washington County, Oregon – Selected Population Profile in the United States (Hispanic or Latino (of any race))." Accessed August 24, 2015. http://www.agcensus.usda.gov.

United States Department of Agriculture, Economic Research Service. 2014a. "Food Away From Home." Accessed December 30, 2014. http://www.ers.usda.gov/topics/food-choices-health/food-consumption-demand/food-away-from-home.aspx.

United States Department of Agriculture, Agricultural Marketing Service. 2014b. "Food Deserts." Accessed December 20, 2014. http://apps.ams.usda.gov/fooddeser5/15 ts/fooddeserts.aspx.

United States Department of Agriculture (USDA). 2012. "Census of Agriculture, 2012." Accessed August 24, 2015. http://agcensus.usda.gov/Publications/2012/Full_Report/Volume_1,_Chapter_1_US/usv1.pdf.

United States Federal Trade Commission. 2012. *A Review of Food Marketing To Children and Adolescents, Follow-Up Report.* Washington, DC: Federal Trade Commission. Accessed June 25, 2015. https://www.ftc.gov/sites/default/files/documents/reports/review-food-marketing-children-and-adolescents-follow-report/121221foodmarketingreport.pdf.

United States Food and Drug Administration. "How to Understand and Use the Nutrition Facts Label." Accessed March 9, 2015. http://www.fda.gov/Food/IngredientsPackagingLabeling/LabelingNutrition/ucm274593.htm.

Useem, John. 1950. "Structure of Power in Palau." *Social Forces* 29(2): 141–48.

Vartanian, L. R. 2010. "'Obese People' vs. 'Fat People': Impact of Group Label on Weight Bias." *Eating and Weight Disorders* 15(3): 195–8.

Vartanian, L. R. and J. Fardouly. 2014. "Reducing the Stigma of Bariatric Surgery: benefits of providing information about necessary lifestyle changes." *Obesity* 22(5): 1233–37.

Vartanian, L. R. and J. Fardouly. 2013. "The Stigma of Obesity Surgery: Negative Evaluations Based on Weight Loss History." *Obesity Surgery* 23(10): 1545–50.

Vlasich, James A. 2005. *Pueblo Indian Agriculture.* Albuquerque: University of New Mexico Press.

Volger, S., M. L. Vetter, M. Dougherty, E. Panigrahi, R. Webb, J. G. Thomas, D. B. Sarwer and T. A. Wadden. 2012. "Patients' Preferred Terms for Describing Their Excess Weight: Discussing Obesity in Clinical Practice." *Obesity* 20(1): 147–50.

Wadden, T. A. and E. Didie. 2003. "What's in a Name? Patients' Preferred Terms for Describing Obesity." *Obesity Research* 11(9): 1140–46.

Waitzkin, H. 1989. "A Critical Theory of Medical Discourse: Ideology, Social Control, and the Processing of Social Context in Medical Encounters." *Journal of Health and Social Behavior* (30): 220–39.

Walinga, David. 2010. "Agricultural Policy And Childhood Obesity: A Food Systems and Public Health Commentary." *Health Affairs* 29(3): 405. doi: 10.1377/hlthaff.2010.0102.

Wann, M. 1998. *Fat! So? Because you don't have to apologize for your size.* Berkley, CA: Ten Speed Press.

Warholm, C., A. Marie Oin, and M. Råheim. 2014. "The Ambivalence of Losing Weight After Bariatric Surgery." *International Journal of Qualitative Studies on Health and Well-being* 9: 22876.

Warin, M, V. Moore, T. Zivkovic, and M. Davies. 2011. "Telescoping the Origins of Obesity to Women's Bodies: How Gender Inequalities are Being Squeezed Out of Barker's Hypothesis." *Annals of Human Biology* 38(4): 453–60.

Weitzman, P. F., A. E. Caballero, A. Millan-Ferro, A. E. Becker, and S. E. Levkoff. 2013. "Bodily Aesthetic Ideals among Latinas with Type 2 Diabetes: Implications for Treatment Adherence, Access, and Outcomes." *Diabetes Education* 39(6): 856–63.

Whiteford, Michael B. 1992. "From Gallo Pinto to Jack's Snacks: Observations on Dietary Change in a Rural Costa Rican Village." *Ecology of Food and Nutrition* 27(3–4): 207–18.

Wiedman, D. 2012. "Native American Embodiment of the Chronicities of Modernity: Reservation Food, Diabetes, and the Metabolic Syndrome among the Kiowa, Comanche, and Apache." *Medical Anthropology Quarterly* 26(4): 595–612.

Williams, Simon N., and Marion Nestle. 2015. "'Big Food': Taking a Critical Perspective on a Global Public Health Problem." *Critical Public Health* 25(3): 245–47.

Willis, M. and K. Waddington. 2013. "Communities of History and Fiction: Re-Investigating Illness Narratives." *Narrative Future for Healthcare Conference.* King's, London.

Wilson, Caroline. 2010. "'Eating, Eating is Always There': Food, Consumerism and Cardiovascular Disease. Some Evidence from Kerala, South India." *Anthropology & Medicine* 17(3): 15. doi: 10.1080/13648470.2010.526699.

Wilson, K. M. and D. W. Satterfield. 2007. "Where Are We to Be in These Times? The Place of Chronic Disease Prevention in Community Health Promotion." *Public Health Research, Practice, and Policy* 4(3): 1–4.

Wolf, N. 1990. *The Beauty Myth: How Images of Beauty are Used Against Women.* New York: Vintage.

World Bank. "Bolsa Família: Changing the Lives of Millions in Brazil" Accessed January 2, 2015. http://go.worldbank.org/3QI1C7B5U0.

World Health Organization (WHO). 1996. World Food Summit. "Rome Declaration on World Food Security & World Food Summit Plan of Action."

World Health Organization (WHO). 2011. NCD Country Profiles. edited by World Health Organization.

World Health Organization (WHO). 2014. BMI Classification. Accessed June 1, 2015. http://apps.who.int/bmi/index.jsp?introPage=intro_3.html.

World Health Organization (WHO). 2014a. Global Status Report on Noncommunicable Diseases. Geneva, Switzerland: World Health Organization.

Wutich, Amber, G. Ryan, and H. R. Bernard. 2014. "Text Analysis: Qualitative and Quantitative Approaches." In *Handbook of Methods in Cultural Anthropology*. H. R. Bernard and C. Gravlee, eds. Lanham, MD: Altamira Press.

Wutich, Amber, A. Ruth, A. Brewis, and C. Boone. 2014. "Social Bonds, Stigmatized Neighborhoods, and Health." *Medical Anthropology Quarterly*. In press.

Yates-Doerr, Emily, and Megan Carney. 2015. "Demedicalizing Health: The Kitchen as a Site of Care." *Medical Anthropology*. Accessed August 21, 2015. doi:10.1080/01459740.2015.1030402.

Young, Lisa R., and Marion Nestle. 2002. "The Contribution of Expanding Portion Sizes to the US Obesity Epidemic." *American Journal of Public Health* 92(2): 246–49.

Young, T. K. 2007. "Are the Circumpolar Inuit Becoming Obese?" *American Journal of Human Biology* 19(2): 181–9.

Yukawa, Keiko, Yoshihiko Yamazaki, Yuki Yonekura, Taisuke Togari, Fusae K. Abbott, Meiko Homma, Minjeong Park, and Yumi Kagawa. 2010. "Effectiveness of Chronic Disease Self-Management Program in Japan: Preliminary Report of a Longitudinal Study." *Nursing & Health Sciences* 12(4): 456–63.

Zhang, Jianjun, Ishwori B. Dhakal, Zijin Zhao, and Lang Li. 2012. "Trends in Mortality from Cancer of the Breast, Colon, Prostate, Esophagus, and Stomach in East Asia: Role of Nutrition Transition." *European Journal of Cancer Prevention* 21(5): 480–89.

Index

About the Contributors

Moya L. Alfonso, Ph.D. is an assistant professor in the Department of Community Health Behavior and Education at the Jiann-Ping Hsu College of Public Health, Georgia Southern University and a prevention fellow for the Florida Prevention Research Center at the University of South Florida. Dr. Alfonso's research interests include adolescent health, physical activity and obesity prevention, community-based participatory research and evaluation, addiction and recovery, and chronic disease self-management. She has managed multiple large scale evaluations of community-based prevention marketing campaigns.

Sara Arias-Steele, M.S. is a doctoral candidate in the Department of Applied Anthropology at the University of South Florida. Her research applies a biocultural approach to the role of adolescent agency and body image perception on eating habits and physical activity among Latinos in Tampa Bay. She co-authored with Dr. David Himmelgreen a community-based participatory research student manual. She was also the Health Project Coordinator for a CBPR Health-Assessment project in Wimauma, Florida with the Hispanic Services Council of Tampa Bay.

Emily Bissett has a Bachelor's of Science degree in nutrition science with minors in Spanish and nonprofit studies from North Carolina State University in Raleigh, North Carolina. She is currently a nonprofit management and global health fellow at Timmy Global Health in Indianapolis, Indiana. She has conducted research in Raleigh, North Carolina, Costa Rica, and the Dominican Republic. Her research interests involve maternal and young child nutrition and food security. Ultimately, Emily plans to complete her doctoral degree in maternal and child public health.

Amy Borovoy, Ph.D. (associate Professor, Princeton University). Borovoy is an anthropologist whose work explores social democracy in Japan with a focus on gender, health, and medicine. Her first book *The Too-Good Wife: Alcohol, Codependency, and the Politics of Nurturance* (University of California Press), addressed the problem of men's heavy drinking and the language of "codependency" as it has been interpreted in urban health care clinics. Borovoy has also written on eating disorders in Japan and the psychiatry of hikikomori youths (young adults who refuse to leave their home). She is currently working on a book manuscript, *Japan in American Social Thought.*

Alexandra Brewis (Slade) Ph.D. is president's professor and director of the School of Human Evolution and Social Change at Arizona State University. She also co-directs the Mayo Clinic-ASU Obesity Solutions initiative, using social science to translate anti-obesity efforts into solutions that work for real people in the real world. Trained as a medical and biological anthropologist (PhD 1992, Arizona), she has lead major field-based projects in the Pacific islands, Mexico, and the U.S. Currently she is conducting a global study of weight-related stigma, examining why its health impacts are spreading and deepening. She teaches in ASU's Global Health and Anthropology degree programs.

Sean Bruna, Ph.D. is an assistant professor of medical anthropology at Western Washington University and uses mixed-methods to examine the intersections of identity and chronic disease. A practitioner of community passed participatory research, Sean's work seeks to reconceptualize "translational theory" as applied with indigenous communities.

Constanza Carney holds a B.A. in anthropology from the University of Florida. She is currently working as a research associate at the UF Department of Emergency Medicine and is committed to improving health outcomes for medically underserved populations in both the hospital and community settings. Her research interests involve health literacy, food security, and HIV. Ms. Carney is pursuing a graduate certificate in global health at UNC Gillings School of Global Public Health and plans to continue her studies in the field of Public Health.

Jose B. Rosales Chavez, M.P.H is a doctoral student at Arizona State University working on topics related to obesity. Some of his areas of interest include analyzing the relationship between body image, obesity and health.

Colleen O'Brien Cherry, Ph.D. is an assistant research scientist and the director of undergraduate programs in the Center for Global Health at the

University of Georgia. As a cultural-medical anthropologist, Dr. Cherry uses qualitative research methods to study culture and meaning in health and medicine, comparative health systems, and social disparities in health.

Lillie Dao received her B.A. in anthropology from the University of Central Florida and masters of public anthropology degree from American University. She is a public anthropologist whose work focuses on intersections of the biological, social, and cultural contexts of health disparities. She has a depth of experience with community-based participatory research focused on issues of social justice, human rights, and health equity. Particularly, she has conducted fieldwork to address issues related to food insecurity, health-care access, maternal-child health, and educational quality.

Merrill Eisenberg, Ph.D., an applied anthropologist, has been involved in policy development and community change in the U.S. for the past 35 years, working on issues including maternal and child health, sexual health and reproduction, community health planning, disability rights, tobacco use, and most recently, the obesity epidemic. Dr. Eisenberg became involved in land use and planning issues in 2010 as part of an obesity prevention project. Since retiring in March 2012, Dr. Eisenberg has continued her involvement in this project on a voluntary basis.

Margaret Everett, Ph.D. is dean of graduate studies at Portland State University. She is a medical anthropologist with a background in Latin American studies. She has conducted fieldwork in Colombia, Mexico and the United States. Recent research includes projects on diabetes care in Oaxaca, Mexico, and community-based health promotion with Latinos in Oregon.

Stevenson Kuartei, M.D. A born and raised Palauan, Dr. Kuartei received his MD degree from the University of Hawaii, trained in family medicine at the University of California, Irvine, and received a post-graduate certificate in public health from the Fiji School of Medicine. He is former minister of health of the Republic of Palau and is currently working in private practice, starting a fellowship in integrative medicine with Arizona Center for Integrative Medicine, and forming a non-profit and non-governmental organization called the Palau Health Foundation.

Alexandra G. Lancey is a graduate student in applied anthropology at the University of South Florida. She has a B.A. in Sociology from Roanoke College. She has conducted work in the southeastern U.S. and the Republic of Palau. Her research interests include childhood obesity and nutrition, environmental education, school-based health promotion, and school and community gardening.

John (Juan) S. Luque, Ph.D. is an associate professor in the Department of Public Health Sciences in the College of Medicine at the Medical University of South Carolina in Charleston. Dr. Luque's research interests are in community-based participatory research, cancer health disparities in minority and underserved communities, community-academic partnerships, and increasing access to cancer prevention and screening through community health worker programs.

Zuhra Malik works as a civil engineer in Baltimore. She graduated from Virginia Tech with a civil engineering degree in May 2015. Her interests lie in people and the built environment, sustainable design, and public health. She speaks Farsi and Spanish.

Chad T. Morris, Ph.D. is associate professor of anthropology and director of the Honors Program at Roanoke College. An applied medical anthropologist, he focuses on means of improving community participation and dissemination of ideas in public health promotion. His current research agenda includes investigating community-driven means of increasing food security and reducing rates of heart disease, diabetes, and obesity in the Republic of Palau.

Elizabeth Serieux is a St. Lucian—American with a deep passion for public health and in particular, global health. Ms. Serieux holds a bachelor of science degree from the St. Francis Xavier University in Nova Scotia, Canada and a master's degree in health policy from the University of Georgia. She is currently a PhD candidate and teaching assistant in the Department of Health Promotion and Behavior, at the University of Georgia.

Stacy Sobell, M.P.H. is farm to school manager at Ecotrust, in Portland, Oregon. Ecotrust is an organization dedicated to building a robust regional food system in the Pacific Northwest. Ecotrust's Farm to School program connects family farmers with schools and other institutions.

Yelena N. Tarasenko, Ph.D. is an assistant professor in the Departments of Health Policy and Management and Epidemiology in the Jiann-Ping Hsu College of Public Health at Georgia Southern University. Dr. Tarasenko's research interests are in cancer prevention and survivorship and behavioral modifications in health disparities populations including rural, Appalachian, and more recently, Hispanic.

Alejandro Tecum is a program director for Adelante Mujeres in Forest Grove, Oregon, where he initiated the Adelante Agricultura program. The Adelante Agricultura program provides aspiring Latino farmers and gardeners with the training and skills necessary to grow produce using sustainable methods and to successfully market their products.

Sarah Trainer, Ph.D. is a post-doctoral research fellow affiliated with Obesity Solutions, a joint initiative between Mayo Clinic and Arizona State University. She completed a Ph.D. in medical and biocultural anthropology at the University of Arizona in 2013. Her research interests focus on food and nutrition, obesity, body image, and stigma in contexts of rapidly increasing rates of obesity and associated chronic diseases on the one hand, and fat stigma on the other. Geographically, she has worked extensively in the Middle East and the American Southwest. Currently, she is conducting research within the bariatric program at Mayo Clinic, focusing on the ways in which stigma affects people pre- and post-surgery.

Deborah Williams, Ph.D., R.N. is a cultural anthropologist and associate director of Mayo Clinic-ASU Obesity Solutions. Her research focuses on the centrality of place and personhood in cultural identity, health and social practice. Her most recent work has focused on understanding the ecological, social and cultural dynamics of health in underserved community populations with an eye to formulating sustainable solutions to our most pressing health issues.

Amanda Wolfe is a sophomore undergraduate student at Roanoke College in Salem, Virginia, majoring in sociology and international relations with a concentration in anthropology. She has contributed toward research and fieldwork focusing on non-communicable diseases in the Republic of Palau. She plans to work in international development after graduation.

Sarah Womack, B.A. is a recent Roanoke College graduate with a degree in biology and a concentration in health care delivery. During her undergraduate career she was involved in research on nutrition-related non-communicable diseases in the Republic of Palau. In the future, she hopes to pursue a career in public health.

Amber Wutich, Ph.D. is a faculty member of Arizona State University's anthropology and global health programs. She has been awarded the Carnegie CASE U.S. professor of the year award for Arizona and ASU's award for excellence in classroom performance. Her research examines the nexus of injustice, resource insecurity, and adaptability, with a focus on water and food in Bolivia, Paraguay, and the U.S. She directs the Global Ethnohydrology Study, a multi-year, cross-cultural study of water knowledge and management. She is associate editor of the journal *Field Methods* and on the faculty of National Science Foundation's research methods programs in cultural anthropology.